Private Practice

Private Practice

*A Handbook
for the Independent
Mental Health Practitioner*

By Robert M. Pressman, Ph.D.

GARDNER PRESS, Inc., New York
Distributed by Halsted Press
Division of John Wiley & Sons, Inc.

New York   London   Sydney   Toronto

GARDNER PRESS, INC.
19 Union Square West
New York 10003

Distributed solely by the Halsted Press Division
of John Wiley & Sons, Inc., New York

Library of Congress Cataloging in Publication Data

Pressman, Robert M
    Private practice.

    1. Psychiatry—Practice. 2. Clinical psycholo-
gy—Practice. 3. Psychiatric social work—Practice.
I. Title. [DNLM: 1. Practice management,
Medical—Handbooks. 2. Psychiatry—Handbooks.
3. Psychology, Clinical—Handbooks. 4. Social
work, Psychiatric—Handbooks. WM21 P935p]
RC440.7.P73   658'.91'61   78-8008
ISBN 0-470-26388-1

PRINTED IN THE UNITED STATES OF AMERICA

To Stephanie, Sarah, and Rebecca

PREFACE

Mental health services are delivered either by public facilities or private practitioners. Public facilities, such as mental health clinics and community and state hospitals, are run by community boards that formulate operational policies. Mental health professionals who work in such a facility are chosen because of their compatibility with its policies. Mental health workers in such facilities are seldom involved in fiscal management or long-range planning.

Very few graduate programs in psychology or psychiatry train the practitioner in the management of mental health services. Management training differs from training in therapeutic skills. The psychiatric resident or psychology intern with several hundred hours of intense case supervision may be ill-prepared for the rigors of private practice. Seldom, if ever, does the intern or resident learn to deal with such problems as developing adequate referral sources, bookkeeping systems, and overhead expenses.

This book deals with ten major themes critical for building, maintaining and expanding private practice in the mental health field. The first four chapters are especially geared to the novice, and the last six provide ample data not only for the novice but also to help the experienced clinician improve and expand his practice. The unique problems of each of the mental health disciplines—social work, psychology and psychiatry—are reviewed in Chapter 9.

The methods discussed in this book might take an individual months or years to discover on a trial-and-error basis. The object of this book is to help the practitioner develop a professionally and financially satisfying practice as quickly as possible.

ACKNOWLEDGMENTS

My grateful thanks is given to the following people and organizations for their help and cooperation in the production of this volume:

The American Psychological Association, The American Psychiatric Association and The National Association for Social Workers for their contribution in the presentation of ethical standards and licensing laws.

Denise Akey and Encyclopedia of Associations for research of professional organizations for private practitioners and Safeguard Business Systems for their assistance in preparing business forms.

Henry Gilfond, Max Faintych, M.D., Norman Orodenker, L.L.D., and S. Richard Sauber, Ph.D., for their advice, counsel and good cheer.

Frank D. E. Jones, M.D. and D. Robert Fowler, M.D. for their contributions on group practice and clinical record keeping.

Acknowledgments

Susan Whitney for her help in typing and preparation of the manuscript.

Gardner M. Spungin, publisher, for his considerable attention to this volume and his commitment to produce it in the finest possible manner.

Stephanie D. Pressman for her support, enthusiasm and editorial input, all of which were deeply appreciated.

R.M.P.

CONTENTS

Contents

Contents

Private Practice

1 PROMISES AND PITFALLS

In this chapter the concept of private practice will be defined and the financial and emotional risks and benefits of establishing a private practice evaluated.

The Lure

Many mental health practitioners have been lured to private practice. Frequently therapists whose principal affiliations are with hospitals or clinics attempt private practice on a part-time basis. Fees of $40 or $50 per hour are more attractive than the salaries earned in public employment. However, despite the promise of greater remuneration many therapists find private practice frustrating and financially disappointing. Some who start private practice give it up or are unable to develop it into a full-time undertaking. Yet, with proper planning, private practice can become a full-time endeavor both financially and emotionally rewarding.

A Definition

Private practice is an arrangement characterized by a *direct contract* between therapist and patient. The therapist is bound by the contract to deliver the highest quality mental health services; the patient is bound to financially compensate the therapist according to a prearranged schedule of fees. In order to implement this arrangement the therapist must establish a setting in which services can be performed, and inform the public of the availability of the services. The practice is conducted in such a manner that successive contracts are secured to produce an ongoing income. The therapist may function as an individual, in a partnership, or as a corporation. In any case, the planning and implementation of the practice, and the rendering of contractual services are the sole responsibilities of the therapist.

The key words in this definition are "direct contract". It is this concept that primarily differentiates private and public practice. The private practitioner having no intervening board or supervisor, is solely responsible for every aspect of service. This special circumstance can be an advantage or disadvantage to the practitioner.

PROMISES AND REALITIES

Private practice is not for everyone, but for some it represents the opportunity for personal and financial growth. In *Establishing and Maintaining a Successful Private Practice* (Lewin, 1978) informal personal inventories help the practitioner assess his fitness for the task. Some of the more obvious advantages and disadvantages of private practice are discussed below. Most therapists who choose private practice anticipate a diversity of patient load, the option of being self-directed, flexibility in working hours and higher pay. While these rewards definitely exist a cautious examination should be made of the realities and the many problems and dilemmas frequently encountered in private practice.

Fluctuating Income

While private practice certainly promises a substantially better income than public practice, the first few years may be marked by financial frustration. It is true that some practitioners become wealthy, but this is the exception to the rule. The private practitioner assumes the entire cost of overhead which includes rent, telephone, insurance and other expenses. In addition, his income tends to fluctuate considerably. In a salaried position, a week's work will render a week's wages. However, in private practice if fees are not collected, it is possible to work an entire week and receive practically no income. In the beginning limited referral sources also contribute to fluctuating income and for the individual used to receiving a regular salary that fluctuation can be very difficult. Although income stabilizes as a practice matures, some fluctuation will always occur.

Isolation

Private practice can be a lonely experience. In a hospital or mental health clinic, the therapist is in contact with co-workers and auxiliary personnel. In private practice, the clinician with no receptionist may spend an entire working day in contact only with his patients.

Multiple Responsibilities

Private practice also requires self-discipline. The practitioner must become completely self-regulated and capable of managing the following responsibilities: proper scheduling of patients, developing referral sources on a continuing basis, collecting fees, paying bills, writing reports, maintaining patients' charts, filing insurance claims, personal-professional development, and providing such benefits to himself as health and life insurance. In order to maintain a healthy practice, all these items must be carefully managed on a day-to-day, week-to-week basis.

Support Services

Consultation and supervisory resources must be established. In private practice the therapist is a primary health care provider and must assume full responsibility for the quality of psychotherapeutic care. No amount of training can prepare the therapist to work effectively in all contingencies. Therefore, he must develop suitable resources to aid him in cases in which his expertise is limited.

Constant Availability

The private practitioner who has sole responsibility for his patients must plan vacations, weekends, and even evenings so his patients have access to emergency treatment. Accessibility may be very difficult to provide for therapists who deal with severely disturbed patients.

Many of these problems can be managed, and even used to the therapist's advantage. Much of the material in the following chapters will help the clinician accomplish this goal. Even with remaining problems, there are definite advantages to private practice.

Control

The private practitioner has considerable control of his office schedule; he may arrange his hours to suit his own style and plans. He, unlike clinic or hospital practitioners, can plan vacations, days off or workshops without the approval of others.

Primary Care Provider

Many clinicians feel that providing primary care for patients from intake to termination is deeply satisfying. Clinics often fragment services into such stages as screening, intake, evaluation and therapy. They may also categorize therapy as child, adult, or marital and assign therapists to specific categories. The independent practitioner has the opportunity to perform a wide range of therapeutic services for a wide range of individuals. Thus, the therapist may eventually establish a practice accommodating the patients and methodologies most suited to his skills and needs.

Direct Payment

The private practitioner is directly paid for his services. Regular, dependable payment constitutes considerable reinforcement for time given to the practice and to the patient. Direct payment, without an institutional middleman, often creates a greater bond between patient and therapist. Continued effort and work in the practice may also result in a considerable increase in income. Many well-managed practices result in very attractive incomes.

LEGAL AND ETHICAL CONSIDERATIONS

Legal Qualifications

Many clinicians complete residencies and interships with little notion of the legal requirements for private practice. Many states have laws governing the rendering of services and the use of various titles. It is critical that an individual wishing to pursue private practice insures that his training will result in licensing, registration, or certification. Licensing is designed to protect the public from individuals blatantly unqualified to practice. All 50 states provide for licensing of physicians and for certification or licensing of psychologists.* 22 states regulate the title and practice of social work.

Although all states have laws which govern or restrict

---

*Certification or licensing of psychologists for private practice is to be differentiated from certification as a school psychologist, which is normally provided by the Department of Education. Certification as a school psychologist is a form of teaching certification applicable only to public school systems.

the private practice of psychotherapeutic and related techniques, they are relatively lenient concerning the practice of such techniques in an institutional or public setting. One rationale for this difference is that private practitioners, who are likely to be unsupervised, require greater regulation than practitioners in public service who are provided with adequate professional supervision. Regulations differ from state to state, usually in two important respects. One type of regulation, certification, addresses the *use of title* by the practitioner; another regulation, licensing, addresses the procedures *performed by* the practitioner. In most states, for example, a person may use the title "psychologist" only after meeting fairly rigid standards. However, in the same states, *functions* performed by psychologists may not be limited to psychologists. Therefore, a person may *practice* psychological techniques in these states as long as he does not call himself a psychologist. Unlicensed vendors in these states often use such terms as "counselor" or "psychotherapist" or any other title not restricted by law. Contrast this with the regulations for physicians; not only is the title "physician" restricted to individuals with very specific training and qualifications, but the *functions* of a physician are also regulated. Only a licensed physician may practice medicine as defined by law.

Ethical Qualifications

Licensing laws barely regulate the delivery of mental health services to the private sector. Physicians may legally practice psychiatry without a psychiatric residency or special licensing. A fully trained psychiatrist, whose residency experience was limited to adults and included virtually no supervision in child therapy, is permitted to practice with children.

Although the title "psychiatrist" does not necessarily convey a specific therapeutic subspecialization, it is less of a generic term than "psychologist" or "social worker". Experimental psychologists, for example, may acquire the certification "psychologist," which in some states will permit them to practice clinical psychology, a field involving completely different supervised experience than the field in which they were trained. While these situations are not illegal they may be considered unethical. Because of inadequate state laws the onus of ethical regulation of psychotherapeutic practice has fallen upon such organizations as the American Psychiatric Association, the American Psychological Association and the National Association of Social Workers.*

These national associations have created boards to examine applicants in their respective fields (see Appendix) and certify their fitness to practice. While in many states, certification is usually considered sufficient evidence for licensing, no state *requires* such certification. The National Register of Health Service Providers in Psychology was formed in 1975 to determine the fitness of psychologists for private practice. It has addressed itself to the problem of differentiating fully trained health service psychologists and academic, experimental, and other non-health service-oriented psychologists. To deal with similiar issues, NASW recently formulated a National Register of Social Workers.

The lack of public regulation places a particularly great responsibility on the individual practitioner for adhering to the ethical standards of his profession. Current regulations primarily restrict the use of specific titles and serve to prevent obviously unqualified individuals from referring to themselves as "psychologist," "psychiatrist" and "social worker." But the private practitioner must constantly re-evaluate his own skills in relation to the needs of the population he serves.

---

*These organizations have published ethical standards for their members (see Appendix) and have formed committees to instruct membership and investigate infractions. Adherence to their standards is necessary for continued membership in these societies.

EVALUATING RISKS AND REWARDS

Staying Solvent

The most difficult problem for beginning practitioners (and experienced ones as well) is predicting income. This raises many questions: Should part-time or full-time employment be considered during the building of one's practice? When is such employment no longer necessary? How long will it take a practice to earn 20, 30, or 40 thousand dollars a year? Answering to these questions avoids unnecessary risks. The experience of other practitioners provide valuable guidelines. Most therapists agree that it takes four to five years to establish a stable practice. Younger practices, tend to be financially vulnerable because they are dependent upon a limited number of perhaps unpredictable referral sources. Income may be limited, therefore, in the first year, and particularly the first few months, of practice. Futhermore, billing and reimbursement procedures sometimes delay receipt of income from 6 to 8 weeks. Unless 6 or 8 months anticipated salary is accessible, some form of supplementary income must be considered in the beginning phases of the practice. Novices may be tempted to begin private practice without sufficiently considering the financial ramifications. It is critical to remember that income not earned is income lost. If the practitioner must borrow money to maintain his living standard, that money will have to be paid back with interest. The financial picture is more encouraging if the clinician is employed at a clinic, hospital, or university while building his practice.

Full-Time vs. Part-Time Employment

The question of full-time or part-time employment arises from the conflict between the need for sufficient time to develop, maintain, and expand the practice and time to supplement income. It is seldom necessary to devote 40 hours a week to beginning a private practice. A minimum of 15 to 20 hours a week will be needed to see patients, do paperwork, and develop referral sources. After perhaps three or four years, less time will be needed to promote referrals. Although some individuals with full-time jobs devote considerable time to developing a practice, this might be at the expense of recreation or family time. The personal toll for 40 or 50 therapy hours a week would also be considerable.

20 hours of employment each week should provide an economic base and also allow the beginning practitioner sufficient hours to develop referrals and provide a variety of appointment times for prospective patients. There is seldom great demand for the therapist who devotes only a few casual hours a week to private practice. Rather, *the commitment to private practice must almost always precede the demand for the therapist's services*. Some risk-taking, therefore, is inevitable. However, if proper precautions are taken regarding office location, overhead control, and other preliminary steps outlined in the following chapters, reasonable risk-taking can be rewarding.

How Many Hours are Needed?

In order to determine necessary supplementary income, it must be learned how many patient hours are needed to derive a particular income and the length of time needed to establish a given number of patient hours. A formula for determining patient hours needed for a desired gross income may be calculated by dividing the weekly gross by the therapist's hourly rate and multiplying by 1.25. The differential of 1.25 should accommodate cancelled appointments and bad debts. If, for example, the therapist wishes to gross $600 a week, at an hourly charge of $40, it would be necessary to schedule approximately 19 hours a week or $\frac{600}{40} \times 1.25 = 19$ (approximately). The 19 hours does not allow time for developing referral sources or doing paperwork. If the same therapist had a part-time job paying $300 a week, 8 or 9 therapy hours would be necessary to meet the $600 goal. Table 1-1 provides a breakdown of hours and fees needed to achieve various income levels based on this formula.

Table 1-1—Hours Needed to be Scheduled Per Week to Derive Target Income

Weekly Income—Adjusted for Cancellations and Poor Collections	Number of Hours Scheduled at Varied Hourly Rates			
	$30/hr.	$35/hr.	$40/hr.	$45/hr.
$200	8.5	7	6	5.5
300	12.5	11	9.5	9
400	16.5	14	12.5	11
500	21	18	15.5	14
600	25	21.5	19	17
700	30	25	22	20
800	33	28.5	25	22

Examination of Table 1-1 reveals the significance of the hourly rate. For example, the practitioner who charges $30 per hour will have an adjusted gross income of $600 for 25 hours work, while the practitioner who charges $40 per hour will have an adjusted gross income of an adjusted gross income of $700 for 22 hours work.

How long will it take?

There are several factors in the length of time needed to acquire a patient load. The therapist who specializes in short term therapy will need a greater number of referrals than the therapist who specializes in long term therapy. The number of a therapist's referrals will depend largely on the amount of time the therapist devotes to developing referral sources. It is difficult for the beginner particularly to predict how long it will take to receive a specific number of referrals. It is not uncommon for the beginning practitioner to have an inflated impression of possible potential referrals. A meeting with a referral source is almost always pleasant and often results in a statement of the source's intended referral. How-

ever, such a referral may take weeks or months to material-
ize. If a potential referral source has a pattern of referring
individuals elsewhere, that pattern is not likely to be soon
changed.

Table 1-2 may be helpful in calculating the length of
time it will take to develop a practice involving 20 patient
hours per week. The numbers are based on anecdotal reports of therapists in private practice. Although it lacks
scientific validity, since every therapist's situation is essentially unique, the chart may serve as a guideline.

Table 1-2—Acquisition of Patient Load

Month	Referrals per month	Total patient hours scheduled by the week	Rate of attrition[1]	Net patient hours by the week[2]
1	2	2	0	2
2	2	3	1	2
3	2	4	1	3
4	3	6	1	4
5	3	8	1	6
6	4	10	2	8
7	3	12	1	9
8	4	15	1	11
9	3	16	2	12
10	4	19	1	14
11	3	21	1	16
12	4	23	2	17
13	3	24	2	18
14	4	27	1	20

[1]Allowance for patients terminating therapy.

[2]Based on addition of referrals less attrition and cancellation at the rate of 25% per week.

Predicting Income

Having developed a basis for predicting patient load
and gross income, the next step is to determine net income
(income remaining after deducting overhead and taxes). Table 1-3 provides a basis for computing gross and net income
in relation to scheduled patient hours. Frequently, overhead
is computed as a percentage of the gross income on the theo-

ry that, as income increases, so do such expenses as secretarial services, supplies, and telephone usage. However,
for the first few months, it is not realistic to use a percentage
formula because such items as rent, basic telephone service
and amortization of expense for office furnishing must be
paid even if no patients are seen. The chart below uses a
figure of 22% of gross income to determine overhead, with a
minimum monthly cost set at $275. This cost is not terribly
high particularly for those practicing in urban locations.
Methods of limiting overhead expenses are discussed in
Chapter 2.

Table 1-3—Weekly Expected Income in First Year of Private Practice

Month	No. Patient Hrs. Scheduled per week	Fees Collected at $40 (Adj. per Fig. 1–2)	Net After Overhead of $275 or 22% of Gross	Weekly Net After Taxes at 22%*
1	2	80	11	9
2	3	80	11	9
3	4	120	26	20
4	6	160	91	71
5	8	240	171	134
6	10	320	250	195
7	12	360	280	219
8	15	440	343	268
9	16	480	374	292
10	19	560	437	340
11	21	640	499	389
12	23	680	530	413

*This approximate figure includes Federal and State income taxes and Social Security tax. The actual figure will vary with changes in number of dependents, state and city taxes and with other sources of income.

Conflict of Interest

It is apparent from examining Table 1-3 that it is almost
imperative for the private mental health practitioner to supplement his income *at least* during the first year of practice.
In supplementing his income, the private practitioner who
works at both a private and public job may be exposing him-

self to a possible conflict of interest. Some care will be necessary to prevent such conflicts, as the following will illustrate. A therapist sees a patient at a mental health clinic 75 minutes from the patient's home. However, the therapist's private office happens to be located a few minutes from the patient's home. If the therapist suggests that the patient be seen at his private office, thus saving him considerable travel time, the therapist is guilty of conflict of interest. No matter what his intentions, if the therapist refers the patient to himself, he is utilizing the clinic to promote his own private practice.

The conflict may be even more subtle. While at the clinic, the therapist might receive a call from his answering service concerning an urgent message from one of his private patients. Returning that call on clinic time involves receiving clinic wages while dealing with a private practice matter. A conflict of interest is involved unless that time is compensated to the clinic in some way. In some cases the matter is difficult to resolve. Some clinicians report that clinic or hospital staff are sometimes sensitive to or even jealous of their private practice endeavors and unless attention is given to avoiding conflicts of interest, misunderstandings occur. Keeping a log of calls and time owed can help allay problems. Also, use of a telephone credit card assures that toll calls do not appear on a clinic's or hospital's bill.

Whether or not the facility has rules governing such conflicts, it is important for the practitioner to have his own strict standard. Referrals to the therapist's own practice must not occur unless the situation is extraordinary and has been fully discussed with the director of the facility. This should apply to patients who themselves ask the therapist to be seen privately. Even if a facility's policy is lenient in this regard, such a practice is likely to be resented by the professional community at large.

Total Involvement

Eventually a practice will increase so that the therapist considers leaving his salaried job. Ideally, at that point, the private practice income should be double the salaried income, but that goal is not always realistic. It would be "safe" to resign a salaried position when at least 20 patient hours had been scheduled for 6 consecutive weeks. The 6 week period is a long enough time to demonstrate a definite trend in the practice. Although the practice might take a temporary dip, the added incentive and excitment of full-time practice would help quickly to recover that loss of revenue.

2

FIRST THREE STEPS

The process of starting a private practice is so elementary that at first glance it may appear simplistic. Nevertheless, each step must be executed successfully in order for a private practice to thrive. The steps will be discussed in detail so that the beginner can learn to establish a successful practice and the experienced therapist can evaluate his own methods against these. The 5 fundamental steps in establishing a thriving practice are:

1. Determining office location;
2. Selecting an office;
3. Furnishing the office in a way that is consistent with your personality, treatment methodology, and budget;
4. Purchasing, equipment, supplies and services necessary for operation;
5. Cultivating referral sources.

In this chapter the first 3 steps will be discussed in detail.

Office equipment, supplies, and services will be reviewed in Chapter 3. Developing referral sources, one of the most essential aspects of both young and mature practices, will be discussed in Chapter 4.

SELECTING LOCATION

While the effect of location on the development of a new practice is important, it can be overestimated. An office in a prestigious medical building will not automatically result in referrals. A poor location, however, can have a deleterious effect which may be difficult or impossible to overcome. A remote area or an area oversaturated with mental health practitioners may be a real hinderance to the beginning practitioner. Most practitioners work in urban areas. The choice of building or section in a large urban center is as important as the choice of town or suburb in a less populous area. The specific setting is also important. For example, in a suburb or small town, patients sensitive about their privacy may be reluctant to park in front of an office whose sole occupant is the therapist.

Finding the best location requires a mixture of art and some science, not unlike psychotherapy itself. An energetic and competent beginner can open a practice almost anywhere a potential clientele exists. The seasoned practitioner, whose referrals are insufficient, perhaps should re-examine his current location. While there are no hard and fast rules for selecting a location, there are some guidelines to consider.

Oversaturation

Most experienced clinicians recommend avoiding areas oversaturated with mental health practitioners. Essentially that means avoiding locations where the supply of practitioners exceeds the demand for their services. In such locations, referral sources are usually well-tapped, hospital staff membership may be closed, and civic groups sufficiently supplied with speakers on mental health. Oversaturation in one's particular discipline is especially critical. A town of 65,000 might support a few practitioners, but not if they all perform only sex therapy.

It may be difficult to determine the precise ratio of demand for services and the availability of practitioners in a given area, but it is possible to make an educated guess. Some state departments of mental health or mental hygiene conduct periodic surveys of availability and demand. These reports frequently provide considerable detail concerning types of services available, including inpatient and outpatient care. Although the number of private practitioners in an area is usually not included, these reports still may be helpful since private clinicians usually are concentrated near hospitals or comprehensive mental health clinics. Professional associations at either the state or regional level often have data concerning the extent of private services or can refer one to somebody who has that information.

A candid private practitioner can often provide considerable information about the potential for practice in his area or in other areas he himself may have considered.

Directors of mental health clinics are usually very knowledgeable concerning services in their geographic area. They frequently know many private clinicians, and also have an idea of the area's potential increased demand for mental health services. Often a call from a private clinician interested in opening a practice, results in an appointment with the clinic's director. Since clinics are frequently interested in developing psychiatric resources, such a contract may develop into a productive professional relationship.

Contact with the administrators of the local hospitals usually produces similar results. They can also provide information about a hospital's departments of psychology, psychiatry, or social work and the availability of staff openings.

17

Urban vs. Suburban

Urban centers offer many advantages for establishing a practice. Certain sections are clearly identified with professional health services and people are accustomed to traveling to these centers which sometimes have a prestige suburban areas lack. Their many hospitals, physicians, public and private schools, lawyers, and civic organizations are all potential referral sources. However, the disadvantages of urban locations must also be considered: office rental is often expensive and, as previously mentioned, the area may be saturated with well-established mental health practitioners. A therapist who lives in or near an urban center will probably not explore office possibilities in distant suburban communities. It makes the most sense for him to find the best site near his home. However, if he has some mobility, greater care can be taken in chosing the site.

It is not mandatory to gravitate to urban areas. Most practices draw from a 5-mile radius and suburban practices frequently extend 20 miles in a particular direction provided highways are adequate. A good compromise, therefore, is to locate in a suburban area en route to an urban area. Rentals are generally lower, traffic less congested, and the route well known or well travelled by most potential clients. Another possibility to consider is locating in a growing community that has few, if any, private mental health practitioners. If the community is adjacent to a metropolitan area, one can probably quickly develop referral sources in the community itself and also draw from the more sophisticated adjacent area. For example, one psychiatrist developed a very successful practice by locating his office in a small New England town bordered by three thriving suburban communities and two hospitals. He not only benefited by referrals from the town education department and local physicians, but also formed affiliations with both hospitals. Fortunately, his office was located on Main Street. No matter how obscure the town, few people worried about finding Main Street.

Established practitioners may be helpful in appraising

the potential in a particular area. Meetings with such referral sources as physicians, lawyers, or certain school personnel (see Chapter 4) also can be helpful. Often these professionals are aware of less well known but potentially competitive mental health resources.

Choice of private practice location can be made before completing a residency or internship program along with preparation for securing an institutional position. The resident or intern who decides to practice in the community where he trains can lay considerable groundwork by developing rapport with a myriad of potential referral sources and exploring suitable office sites while completing training.

Cost Saving Considerations

Aside from paying salaries, office rental is the practitioners single biggest expense. The two strategies most frequently used involve utilizing the home or the university as an office site.

House as the Office. Utilizing part of one's house or apartment as an office reduces the cost of rental and eliminates the cost of travel to and from work. But unless one's home is located in a suitable area, the savings will be more than offset by difficulty in attracting clientele. Referral sources may also interpret a home office as lack of personal and financial commitment to the practice. Some practitioners, however, do conduct successful home practices. It is traditional in most communities to permit doctors to utilize their houses for their offices even in a strictly residential area. In an apartment building, a lease might restrict such use. If a home is poorly located, it might be utilized as a second office after the practice is more established.

A home can be used satisfactorily as an office if an effort is made to preserve the office's professional identity. It is preferable for one's home to appear to be at the office rather than the office at one's home. The entrance and sign should be arranged so that the patient enters the office or waiting room rather than the portion of the house or apartment used by the family.

Second Office. A practitioner with a spacious home may want to utilize some part of it as a *second* office. If the home is a substantial distance from the primary office, it gives the practitioner the opportunity to see patients from a different geographic area. Also, practitioners who work with depressed, suicidal patients and who plan to provide crisis sessions may find it more convenient to meet clients at home rather than travel to another location, especially late at night

Home offices located in strictly residential areas are not recommended as principal locations. The address is not likely to convey serious private practice intent to referral sources. Furthermore, patients who have difficulty with intimacy may be reluctant to go to a therapist's home. A therapist who uses a secondary location should indicate the principal office address on his stationery. Also, unless he and his family are well-disciplined, there will probably be interference between family and practice. Business time and family time may both suffer.

University Office. While it is tempting to use a university office for private practice, it is best to resist the temptation. Even if the university does not object and overhead costs would be greatly reduced, it is a poor place to conduct private practice. The possibility of conflict of interest would be greatly increased, and university colleagues may wonder where one's interests lie and become suspicious or distrustful. Few university academic offices provide adequate waiting areas or for patient privacy. Finally, both patients and referral sources are likely to assume the practice is under university auspices and thus the private practitioner's professional identity would be obscured.

Selecting an Address

An office on a well marked, well known street will be relatively easy for new patients to find. Patients frequently feel considerable anxiety prior to the first visit. Complicated directions may create more ambivalence about keeping the appointment. Getting lost and arriving late will not contribute positively to the first session. Parking is also important. Ample free or inexpensive parking should be available; half-hour or hour meters are not satisfactory. It would be helpful to have the office near bus or subway lines.

It is not necessary to select the most modern building. In fact, some practitioners feel such locations tend to be impersonal and dehumanizing. Of course, a poorly maintained, older building is also a poor choice. The goal should be a pleasant, well-kept, reasonably priced location.

SELECTING THE OFFICE

Rental Cost

If all other things are equal, the final consideration in office selection should be cost. Meeting overhead expenses is one of the most difficult problems facing the beginner. High overhead creates severe financial pressures in the first stages of practice and drains away profits in later stages.

Office rental space is usually discussed in terms of square feet. The cost is computed using the following formulas:

$$\text{Monthly rent} = \frac{\text{No. of sq. ft.} \times \text{Cost per sq. ft.}}{12}$$

or

$$\text{Cost per sq. ft.} = \frac{\text{Yearly Rent}}{\text{No. of sq. ft.}}$$

If space costs $7.00 per square foot, which is about average for professional offices, and 300 feet are needed, the monthly rent will be:

$$\frac{300 \times 7.00}{12} = \$175$$

If the rent is \$200 per month for 300 square feet, the cost per square foot is:

$$\frac{\$2,400}{300} = \$8 \text{ per sq. ft.}$$

Generally, all space wholly occupied by the tenant is computed in the rent. This includes not only the office but closets, bathroom, and, of course, a waiting area, if applicable. Some buildings provide shared waiting areas, as well as toilet facilities, which will be reflected in the office rent. Rentals vary considerably in different sections of the country and according to the particular attributes of each building. Similar offices may cost \$22 per square foot in Manhattan and \$7 per square foot in Cleveland. Also, the cost per square foot may vary according to the number of square feet rented. A 1,500 square foot rental may be less expensive *per foot* than a 100 square foot rental.

Minimum Space Needed

A large office is uneconomical and contributes little to the therapy session. 100 square feet is adequate for individual psychotherapy or therapy with four people including the therapist. A 10 feet by 10 feet area, the size of the average second bedroom, is large enough to accommodate a small livingroom arrangement of a couch, two chairs, and even a small desk and filing cabinet. Less space will result in crowding.

Groups, of course, require more space. A minimum of 200 square feet is necessary to conduct group therapy involving 8 to 10 people. 80 square feet is adequate for therapists' waiting area because, unlike in a dentist's or doctor's office, only one family or patient would usually be waiting at a time.

A waiting area of 100 square feet would also accommodate a secretary or receptionist.

Neighbors

Another factor in choosing an address should be the other tenants. It is preferable, in sharing a building, that the other tenants be health or mental health professionals. Tenants who produce noise, traffic, or other disturbances may serve either to encumber your practice or embarras your patients.

PURCHASING OR LEASING

Purchasing an Office

Most beginning practitioners rent rather than purchase an office, although there are many advantages to purchasing. Real estate value almost always increases with time. Purchase of an office is a good investment and should be considered if one has the financial resources.

However, the purchase of an office has very little to do with the practice itself. It is merely a way of manipulating capital, if you have it.

Leasing

The alternative to purchasing a building or office is renting space either on a month-to-month basis or by lease. A month-to-month rental is less formal. Rent is paid each month, and unless otherwise specified, either party may terminate the agreement by giving sufficient notice according to state business statutes (usually 15 to 30 days). The landlord can also raise the rent at his discretion by giving the same notice.

A lease, on the other hand, is a written agreement which

specifies the responsibilities and obligations of the landlord and tenant including the duration of the rental and the amount of rent. It may also specify such obligations of the landlord as heat, air-conditioning, and hot water supply and such obligations of the tenant as utility payment and cleaning. It is a good idea to have a lawyer examine a lease; his $25 to $50 consultation fee may save money in the end. However, any elements in the lease that need to be negotiated with the landlord, should be done by the tenant rather than his lawyer. If it is going to be that difficult to deal with the landlord, one should look for another place.

A lease is not sacrosanct. It can be altered before it is signed, provided both parties agree to and initial the changes. Above all, one should avoid a "Landlord's Lease" which provides the landlord with many rights and privileges and places the tenant in a precarious position. A lawyer can easily spot a "Landlord's Lease."

A problem can arise when the tenant needs to terminate the lease prior to the end of its duration. Unless otherwise specified, a lease can be assigned (taken over by someone else) or sublet. If, as in some cases, the landlord's permission is required to do this, the lease should state that such permission "will not be unreasonably withheld."

There is some question as to whether a month-to-month rental or a lease is preferable. In most cases the landlord has a preference. If a deposit is entailed, it is essential to have indicated in writing the conditions under which the depost will be returned. In fact, deposits for professional office rental are rarely required. A 12 to 18 month lease is probably reasonable for the beginning practitioner. That period is long enough to test a specific geographic location thoroughly but would not impose a terrible financial obligation should the location prove to be a poor choice. Conversely, the beginning practitioner needs assurance of an unencumbered year or two while he gets established. In addition to assuring uninterrupted rental, a lease protects the tenant from rent increases for its duration.

FURNISHING THE OFFICE

Layout

The layout of the office will depend on the shape of the room; location of doors, closets, windows, and electrical outlets; style of therapy; and, to some degree, financial resources. Of course, special *clinical* orientations or techniques, such as psychoanalysis or biofeedback, may demand specific types of furniture and arrangements.

Cost of Furnishings

Price of furniture varies greatly according to its structure and how it is marketed. In addition to style, some consideration should be given to cleaning, stain and friction resistance, and durability. Waiting room furniture receives the most abuse and should be made of such durable material as wood, metal or high-impact plastic.

The cost of upholstered furniture is principally affected by the type of material used. Folding chairs can usually be purchased for under $10. Stacking chairs, which are constructed of metal with a non-folding, high-impact plastic seat, may be purchased for under $15. They are slightly more attractive than folding chairs. Cushioned wooden or metal chairs will range from $35 to $70, while upholstered chairs will range upwards from $125.

It would be useless to speculate here on the relative cost of different styles of upholstered furniture. An item as conventional as a three-seater couch can range from $200 to $3,000. The same is true of desks. A perfectly adequate executive desk, 30" x 60", can be purchased for under $175 but a solid teak one will obviously cost considerably more.

Basically, furniture should be comfortable, durable, and attractive. Most practitioners prefer a restful, nondistracting office atmosphere. Most important, the office should be a comfortable place for the therapist who will spend most of his time away from home there.

CONSIDERING THE PATIENT

Signs

The purpose of a sign is to help the patient find the office *after* an appointment is made. In some states the use of a sign to advertise one's practice might be considered unethical. Most professional organizations have codes regarding the formulation of signs. The outdoor sign should contain only the therapist's name, his highest degree and, if he chooses, his professional identity, such as psychologist or psychiatrist. In some states, including a telephone number on a sign might result in a call from an ethics committee.

The most important aspect of the sign is its readability. The background should be light, preferably white, with dark preferably black lettering. Wood can be used for the frame, but is too porous for the background because it tends to weather after only a few years. Painted metal prolongs the readability and the life of the sign. This is particularly true if the sign is exposed to the elements.

The sign should be consistent with the format of the community. A professional building may have a special area designated for signs. In cases of uniform signs, the landlord sometimes provides them for a nominal fee. Some communities have ordinances regulating outdoor signs and a permit may be necessary before a sign is legally installed. A practitioner is ordinarily not denied the right to place a discreet sign on his building or lawn, but to do so without first getting a permit may result in unnecessary difficulty and resentment.

Waiting Room

Patients usually like some degree of privacy while waiting for their appointment. If a hall with an outside door is situated between the office and waiting room, a patient can leave the office and avoid making contact with the next patient. On the other hand, if the outside entrance is in the waiting room, patients will pass each other coming and going.

The area itself should be comfortable and stocked with a few *current* magazines. *Time* or *Newsweek*, *Sports Illustrated*, *Ms.*, *Psychology Today* and *People* are a few that patients frequently enjoy. Out-of-date magazines invite negative patient reaction. If children will be using the waiting room, *Seasame Street*, *Electric Company*, and assorted coloring books and crayons are worthwhile choices. Chalk and a small chalk board attached to the wall are unfailingly popular with children.

Some therapists think it pleasant to have hot water with instant coffee or tea available in the waiting room. However, such amenities should be avoided if children will be using the area. In addition to the possibility of scalding or electrical shock, the coffee, tea, and sugar are likely to become objects of a five-year-old's curiosity.

Acoustics

A poorly soundproofed office is a deterrent to therapy. Noise from a busy hallway or a nearby office is distracting and conveys lack of privacy. Of course, sound transmitted from the office constitutes a violation of the patient's right to privacy.

Most sound is transmitted through the door's perimeter. To remedy this universal problem, some therapists purchase sound-resistant doors and frames. This is the most effective method and the most costly. An alternate method is to "winterize" the door with weather stripping. A hardware store can provide advice and materials for such a project. The total cost will probably be under $5. Residual sound will leak through and around the door but can be masked by placing one or two radio speakers in the waiting room and playing music.

Display of Diplomas

An area of the office may be set aside to display diplomas. Diplomas are sometimes lightheartedly referred to as "wallpaper" but in private practice they have a special function. The practitioner must rely on his own reputation rather than the reputation of a clinic or hospital in which he works. The display of appropriate diplomas may be a source of reassurance to some patients, even if they cannot evaluate the importance of each one. It is important, therefore, that diplomas or certificates displayed reflect competency or achievement. Diplomas of graduation and of licensure are appropriate. Appropriateness of certificates of *membership* in professional societies depends upon the qualifications of the society. The American Psychological Association, for example, prohibits members from advertising their membership in any way since membership reflects interest and minimal qualifications rather than competency. On the other hand, membership in the American Society of Clinical Hypnosis requires a demonstration of training and skill, and its diploma would be appropriate for display.

3   SETTING UP THE OFFICE

A good location and an attractive, affordable office are only two of the four basic elements for a successful private practice. The office must become a functioning entity and methodology established to handle patient inquiries, appointment scheduling, and collection.

TELEPHONE SERVICE

The first step in setting up an office is the installation of telephone service. The telephone company requires that business lines be used for business purposes, although some beginners try to reduce costs by attempting to secure residential service. Business service utilizes the same equipment but costs more to install and maintain than residential service. The rationale for the additional cost is that commercial customers use equipment more extensively and require more prompt repair service. A business service customer is entitled to a title (physician, psychologist, etc.) in the directory, a free yellow page listing, and additional paid yellow page listings.

Equipment

A variety of telephone equipment is available but simplicity is important if overhead is to be kept low. An added cost of $25 per month may seem small but would amount to $6,000 over a 20-year period. It is unlikely that a beginning practitioner in a one person office needs more than one telephone line or one instrument. Offices with more than one practitioner or a receptionist obviously need more equipment.

Other Telephone Companies

The Bell Telephone System is not the sole provider of telecommunication hardware and service. Excellent equipment can be rented, leased or purchased from a number of smaller, competitive companies, sometimes at great savings if multiple lines and instruments are involved. In recent years even the major telephone companies have offered customers the opportunity to purchase equipment. Frequently such purchases pay for themselves in 12 to 24 months. The January 1978 *Consumer Reports* provides considerable information on this subject.

TELEPHONE ANSWERING SERVICES AND MACHINES

A Necessity

The first contact a client makes with a therapist's office is probably by telephone. Most therapists are unable to answer the telephone themselves because they are either busy with patients or away from the office. Few individual practices can afford a fulltime receptionist, although small group practices often employ a full-time or part-time receptionist to answer calls. Clients almost always prefer to speak to an office employee rather than an answering service or answering machine, but no office has a 24-hour, seven-day-a-week receptionist. Therefore, every office requires an answering service or machine for some hours in the day. Legally, inaccessibility could lead to a malpractice suit.

Answering Service

When telephone service is installed, the phone company can provide a connection between the clinician's telephone and an answering service switchboard. When the clinician's telephone rings, a light and a sound will signal the switchboard, and, depending upon the therapist's instructions, the switchboard operator will answer the call or not. The best type of service for a clinician is 24-hour 7-day coverage. The minimum cost of an answering service is about $25 a month. Some companies charge a basic monthly fee with an additional charge for calls in excess of 50 or 100.

The advantage of an answering service rather than an answering machine is that most operators are adept at soliciting important information from a caller and can be provided with the names of patients whose telephone calls should be forwarded to the therapist immediately. The critical difference between an answering service and a machine is that the service can locate the therapist in an emergency provided, of course, it has been given sufficient information. Services which cater to medical clientele are recommended over those whose clients are primarily businesses or private individuals. A medically oriented service will more likely be experienced in eliciting appropriate information from callers and dealing with emergencies.

Since it is difficult to select one service over another, one can request a list of clients and call those references in order to evaluate a service. It is unlikely, however, that the service will give out the names of any dissatisfied customers.

Instructions. It takes time for the service and the therapist to learn each other's methods of operation. The service will ask the therapist for his home phone number, other numbers where he can be reached in an emergency, and a set of instructions. These instructions should be as simple as possible. For example, the service could be instructed to answer after the third ring, permitting the therapist not to answer if it is inconvenient. The service can be instructed to call back immediately in the event of an emergency. Two successive calls, therefore, would be interpreted as urgent.

Style. Whatever salutation is used, it is important that the caller know immediately that the service and not an office receptionist is answering the phone. Salutations such as "Answering for Dr. Smith" or "Dr. Smith's answering service" are more appropriate than "Dr. Smith's Office" which might give the impression that the receptionist is answering the phone. Most patients are accustomed to dealing with answering services, but if a caller thinks he is talking with a receptionist, he may try to set up an appointment and become frustrated.

If used properly, the answering service can become a real asset. Professionals frequently feel their service is inadequate in providing or obtaining accurate information, but often the service has to act on incomplete information. If, for example, the therapist wants the service to know that he is going to be at a specific restaurant, it is his responsibility to give the answering service the phone number as well as the name of the restaurant. The service should also be informed when the therapist leaves a specified location.

Checking In. It is important to check with the service reasonably frequently, at least before going to the office in the morning and before retiring at night. It is a good idea to call the service any time after being away from the office during the day. If the service is called when the therapist arrives at and leaves the office, it will be certain of his whereabouts and be able to assure clients that he checks in frequently. This helps alleviate a client's anxiety about when his message will be received.

A therapist in part-time private practice should receive client's calls at his own business number. Except in emergencies, referral sources and clients should not be given his other employment number. Clients or referral sources who regularly reach the therapist at a clinic or hospital are more likely to view him as an employee of that facility than as a serious private practitioner.

Answering Machines

Some clinicians prefer to use an answering machine. The principal advantage of an answering machine is its cost, which ranges from $150 to $400, depending upon features. Some models sell for less than $100, although their quality may be unpredictable.

Some companies permit the consumer to lease an answering machine over a period of one to two years and purchase it at the end of that time for a nominal fee. After the machine is purchased, there will, except for maintenance charges, be no further expense for an answering service.

Some answering machines require special installation which the telephone company may insist on performing. The phone company also may charge a monthly fee for an interconnecting device intended to protect its equipment against damages resulting from incompatibility with the answering machine. Some machines have a built-in interconnecting device that would eliminate the need for the monthly service charge.

Therapist's Message. The following is an example of the type of recorded message a therapist might leave for patients: "This is Dr. Jones answering by recorded message. I will be returning to my office at 1 o'clock. If you leave your name and telephone number at the tone, I will return your call promptly. If this is an emergency, I may be reached at 555-0306." It is more reassuring and more personal for a therapist to use his own voice in the recording than a receptionist's. It is also reassuring for the message to indicate when the therapist will return to the office. Of course, leaving an alternate number is optional.

Some clinicians use both a mechanical and live service, indicating in the recorded message the phone number for the answering service. Use of an alternate number might reduce the possibility of a malpractice claim based on the contention that the therapist was inaccessable.

OFFICE HELP

A clinician alone in practice seldom needs the services of a receptionist. Certainly the beginning clinician does not. Unlike a general practitioner, the typical mental health practitioner sees only one client or one family every half hour to hour and a half and has virtually no need for traffic management. He also has fewer financial transactions and incoming calls than a medical doctor. Since most practitioners correspond regularly with referral sources and periodically provide assessments and reports, they do need a typist. However, it is not always necessary to hire a full-time secretary.

Transcription Services

Transcription services are usually listed under "stenographers" in the yellow pages. They charge a flat rate, either per page, or per typewritten line, including date, address, salutation and closing. Many of these services provide 24 hour telephone access to a dictating machine. Some clinicians use these services, therefore, even if they employ a part-time typist.

34

Unless the transcriber knows the therapist's style well and the therapist enunciates with extraordinary clarity, there are likely to be errors in the transcribed material. Because voice quality is somewhat distorted over the telephone, the dictated material is difficult to discern. Unless the transcription company is nearby or has a delivery service, the delay in mailing a corrected draft will negate the advantage of the service. Also, clinical vocabulary, unless spelled out, might result in such transcription errors as Wexler for Wechsler, Skid Row for schizoid, dish function for dysfunction, etc.

The service must be provided with stationery and, of course, any special typing instructions. If a special format is used for reports, a sample should be given them to keep on hand. As in the case of answering services, instructions should be succinct and demands kept to a minimum.

Secretary

There is an advantage to hiring a part-time secretary, even at the very beginning stages of private practice. This arrangement is more satisfactory than a transcription service because, over a period of time, the secretary can be trained in the therapist's style of work. The mechanics of recruiting and hiring a staff are discussed in Chapter Eight.

STATIONERY

Attention should be paid to the quality of the therapist's stationery since it represents him to his patients, referral sources, and colleagues.

Letterhead

Quality of letterhead stock is expressed in terms of weight and rag content. Average letterhead stock is 20-pound weight, with 16-pound weight appropriate for airmail and when 5 to 6 page letters are the rule rather than the exception. Some corporations use 25-pound weight paper to convey a more substantial image.

Rag content refers to the amount of cotton fiber present in the paper. For private practice a minimum of 25 percent rag content is recommended. Since letterhead is used only for the first page, comparable paper is needed for second and third pages. Good quality paper, with 25 to 50 percent rag content, can be identified by a distinctive manufacturer's watermark which frequently indicates the percent of cotton used.

Letterheads are usually printed on 8½ by 11-inch sheets although smaller sheets may also be obtained.

Copy, or the words printed on the letterhead, should include the therapist's name followed by his highest degree, his profession or speciality, and address and telephone number. A statement about "hours by appointment only" would be more appropriately saved for business cards. The copy on the envelope should be limited to name followed by highest degree, and address. Some patients may be sensitive to having the mailman, or anyone else for that matter, know they are receiving correspondence from a therapist.

Envelopes

Envelopes come in various sizes designated by number. The most common business envelope is #10; return envelopes are #9 envelopes; small billing envelopes are #7. Envelope quality is not as important as letterhead quality but matching envelopes can be printed for a small cost.

Amount of Stationery Needed

The beginning clinician seldom writes more than three to five letters a week for the first several months. The more energetic and experienced practitioner may generate as many as 15 letters a week. Because the greatest expense in printing is typesetting and press preparation, 50 sheets cost nearly as much as 250 sheets. Therefore, a roll of 250 to 500 is recommended. Printing normally takes about a week, unless special paper has to be ordered. A marker placed above the last 50 pieces of stationery will serve as a reminder to reorder.

When material is picked up from the printer, the copy should be checked for printing errors. If the printer has been given a typed or clearly handwritten model, printing errors are his responsibility. In very large orders, the printer may want the customer to check the proofs. Also, the beginning, middle and end of the run should be checked for printing uniformity; and the backs of the envelopes and letterheads should be examined to see if a faint mirror-image of the copy appears. If that happens, the press was either over-inked or the freshly printed material was improperly handled. Such material should be rerun at the printer's expense.

Appointment Cards

Appointment cards are given to patients to indicate the time of their next appointment. They are particularly convenient for appointments not scheduled at a regular weekly time. These cards can be inexpensively printed by offset. In addition to the therapist's name and address, the card includes space to write the date and time of the patient's next appointment. Below is an example of a typical appointment card. Unless these cards are given out routinely, it is unlikely that more than several hundred will be needed.

JANE M. ROBERTS, Ph.D.
PSYCHOLOGIST

30 Liberty Street
Warwick, New York 10990

YOUR NEXT APPOINTMENT

DATE   DAY   TIME

(914) 292-7610

#6 Double Window Envelope (not actual size)

```
David J. Heines, M.D.
One Medical Plaza
Allentown, Minn. 55112



Space for patient's address
```

STATEMENT

For professional services rendered:

12/2/79 Psychotherapy 1 hr $45

Billing Stationery

Sometimes a special letterhead is used for bills or statements, particularly in beginning practices and in smaller practices that log less than ten patient hours a week. The system recommended for larger practices is discussed in Chapter 5. The printing format shown above allows the statement to be mailed in inexpensive windowed envelopes with no additional typing.

Business Cards

Business cards are an inexpensive item useful to have when dealing with referral sources. Some referral sources give patients the therapist's card. A white card stock with black lettering is most frequently used. Cards are usually printed in lots of 250. The copy should provide only essential information about specialty, location and availability. The following is an example of a typical business card.

MARK BENJAMIN, Ph.D.

PSYCHOLOGIST

1313 Blueview Terrace, Ames, Iowa 60735

HOURS BY APPOINTMENT ONLY

(201) 765-4321

TYPEWRITERS

Unless correspondence to be typed is given to a firm or individual with a typewriter, the therapist will have to purchase or rent one.

Electric typewriters designed for commercial use are sturdier and more reliable than most electric portables or manual typewriters. Because commercial typewriters are expensive, it is worth looking for a used machine either at a typewriter store or through the want ads under "Office Equipment."

The more expensive typewriters produce crisp, attractive copy but must get a lot of use to justify their cost. A $600 or $850 typewriter is certainly not a necessity for the beginning practitioner.

Commercial typewriter companies and many typewriter stores offer equipment on lease/purchase or installment plans, which are helpful if capital is limited. An installment plan for equipment over $200 allows the therapist to spread his initial expenses over a period of a year or two.

PHOTOCOPY EQUIPMENT

It is essential to have copies of correspondence for informational and legal purposes. Photocopy equipment which is costly and requires constant maintenance, should be considered only if the therapist's needs exceed 250 copies per month. Few private practices demand that, however, and coin operated copy equipment and services are readily accessible at libraries, universities, some post offices, drug stores, and "instant printing" companies.

Inexpensive table-top photocopy machines, which utilize heat to transfer the copy can be purchased for $200 to $300. However, because supplies are expensive individual copies on such machines cost between 11 and 13 cents, the process is slow, and errors often necessitate re-copying.

One office practice that greatly reduces the need for photocopies is the use of carbons. A disposable carbon pre-fastened to a second sheet costs from one-half to one cent.

DICTATION EQUIPMENT

Dictation equipment properly used can be of enormous value. There may be some difficulty in initial adjustment but eventually productivity will increase considerably. 5 or 6 times more material can be dictated in a given period of time than can be written in longhand.

Type of Equipment

The two basic pieces of dictation equipment are a recorder and a transcriber, which is used for playback of the material to be typed. Often a single piece of equipment contains both features. A separate recorder and transcriber are necessary only if transcription and dictation must occur simultaneously. A portable dictating machine rather than a desk model is advantageous because it is battery-operated and can be used in an automobile. The size, weight and location of controls are critical factors in a portable machine since it must be operated with one hand.

Cost

Dictation equipment varies considerably in cost, with cassette tape models usually the least expensive. First-quality dictation equipment is probably too expensive for the beginning practitioner. In a cassette tape model, the transcriber should be completely operable with a foot pedal in order to free the typist's hands.

FILE CABINETS

An important but often overlooked item is a file cabinet to hold patient charts and other important, confidential matter. A two-drawer cabinet is adequate for the first two years of practice. Three- or four-drawer cabinets tend to be cumbersome and obtrusive. Some cabinets are fairly inexpensive while other fire resistant models cost more than $250. Cabinets should be full size—that is, approximately 25 to 28 inches deep—and have lockable suspended drawers that can be fully rolled out without the threat of the cabinet tipping forward.

Once the office is set for full operation, the most critical step, acquiring patients remains.

4 DEVELOPING REFERRALS

There is no substitute for a good reputation for receiving referrals and developing a practice. Unless good will is established and excellence in one's work demonstrated, advertising and other strategies have limited value. However, unless others are informed of his services, the beginning private practitioner may be idle, despite excellent training and clinical skills. Developing a stable 20- to 30-patient-hour-a-week practice takes an extraordinary degree of effort over a long period of time.

The dilemma confronting many practitioners with several years of postgraduate training are their feelings that it is undignified to indicate to others the wish or need for referrals. One therapist who called on a nursing home to meet the director said he was horrified to realize that, for a moment, he felt the "No Soliciting" sign on the front door applied to him.

However, the process of developing referrals and informing others of one's availability permits other professionals to provide better care for their patients. Many physicians, for example, like to have a reference list of clinicians who provide various types of psychotherapeutic services. A physician who tentatively diagnoses anorexia nervosa would be disinclined to treat such a case himself. The population one is able to service benefits from the known availability of the services.

Also it is not shameful to want to be gainfully employed and provide an income for oneself and family. Developing referral sources is the mainstay of private practice and the income derived from that practice.

INDIRECT CONTACT

Newspaper

Broadest exposure comes from an announcement in a local newspaper. Some practitioners feel this method is too commercial, and some professional organizations flatly prohibit their members from placing such announcements. However, in some communities it is standard practice for a clinician to announce the opening of his practice with a single newspaper notice. It is doubtful that such announcements alone bring referrals, but together with other exposure they have acumulative effect on potential referral sources.

A newspaper notice may also be used to announce a change of address or the addition of an associate. However, if a therapist is contemplating using a newspaper announcement, he should check first with the ethics committee of his local professional organization.

Placing the Announcement. Generally, the announcement should be limited to the therapist's name, highest degree, specific area of specialization, telephone number and address. A typical announcement reads as follows:

> Harry L. Sullivan, Ph.D.
> announces the opening of his office
> for the practice of family and
> child psychology.
> 3180 Bellevue Avenue
> Dockray, Illinois
>
> Telephone 403-555-7038

Placing an announcement in a newspaper can be done by telephone but to avoid the possibility of error, it is worthwhile typing the copy on one's professional stationery and mailing or delivering it to the newspaper's business office.

The size of an advertisement is expressed in column inches. An ad that is 2 inches long and 2 newspaper columns wide is 4 column inches. An announcement should never be more than two columns wide and should not exceed 2 to 3 inches in depth. The newspaper or one's professional organization can probably indicate the customary size of such announcements. In some states the repetition of such an announcement could be construed as unethical advertising and might result in censure by some professional organizations.

Mailed Announcements

Many practitioners like to send attractively printed announcements to colleagues and potential referral sources. The information on the mailed announcement will not vary greatly from the newspaper announcement but has advantages of reaching a carefully selected target population. Also such announcements may possibly be saved and referred to at a later date.

Printing cost will range from 50 to several hundred dollars, depending on the quantity ordered and the printing technique used. This does not include the cost of postage, a mailing list, and addressing envelopes. Such a mailing is itself unlikely to generate referrals but together with other exposure will have a cumulative effect.

An announcement card should be of good quality. The stock, or paper on which the announcement is printed, should be plain white with or without an indented area for the copy.

An announcement can be printed by engraving, letter-press, offset or thermoengraving. Engraving is the best and the most expensive method. Hot type letterpress, which utilizes molten metal to form the type, also gives excellent quality. Photo offset printing, the least expensive method, is seldom recommended for announcements. Thermoengraving uses standard letterpress or offset printing with ink that, when exposed to heat lamps, causes the letters to rise slightly. Thermoengraving is very frequently used since it gives the appearance of engraving at a significantly lower price.

Because the greatest expense in all these methods is in setting up plates and presses, the difference in cost between printing 50 and 200 announcements may be negligible.

Mailing Lists. The mailing list should include the names of all potential referral sources. The telephone directory yellow pages is not a very good source of names because of abbreviations and incomplete addresses but can be used if nothing better is available. Professional organizations frequently provide or sell mailing lists. However, mental health practitioners are not usually considered major referral sources. A physicians mailing list may be obtained by writing to the local chapter of the medical society or by inquiring at local hospitals. If their office addresses are unavailable, announcements can be sent to physicians at the hospital. A mailing list of lawyers can be obtained from the local bar association.

Announcements should be sent to those school personnel who are in position to make referrals, including the principal and vice principal, special education director, director of pupil personnel services, director of guidance, guidance counselors, school psychologist, learning disability teacher, remedial reading teacher, resource teacher, school nurse, social worker and attendance officer. Names and titles of school personnel should be available from the school office. Announcements can be sent to their school addresses or in care of the superintendent's office.

It is inadvisable to send announcements to all teachers since such a flood of mail would give the appearance of soliciting business. Also, sending announcements to all teachers might be viewed as usurping the role of appropriate referral sources.

Directories. A directory of community services, which includes the names of many organizations and the names and addresses of their directors, is often available at public or university libraries. Depending on the size of the community, these references cost between $3.50 and $10 and are an excellent mailing list source. It is always best to address announcements to a specific individual.

Addressing and Mailing. The therapist's return address should be printed on the envelope. Although the post office does not encourage this, it is most attractive to have the return address on the back flap of the envelope. The envelope can be addressed by hand or typed. Address labels are impersonal and give the impression of junk mail. First Class postage, which guarantees the forwarding or return of undeliverable mail, increases the probability of the announcement being opened and read.

Personalized Letter

A concise, personal letter to potential referral sources is another form of indirect contact. Such a letter might read:

> Dear Doctor Stacey:
>
> I recently opened an office on Bridge Street where I will be providing child and adult psychotherapy. I hope these services may be of benefit to some of your patients.
> I would be delighted to meet and discuss these services with you further
>
> Sincerely,

47

If it is impractical for these letters to be typed individually, the body of the letter, typed on the therapist's letterhead, can be printed by offset at a cost of about $6 for 100. When the date, inside address, salutation and signature are added later, the letter will have the appearance of being personally typed.

A business card or an enclosure can be included with the letter. The enclosure, which provides a more detailed description of the therapist's services along with the referral procedure, can be printed on heavy colored stock with a paper offset plate. Figure 4-1 is an example of the type of enclosure that can be used. Before printing, the stock and envelope should be weighed to be certain that the mailing is under one ounce, to reduce postage costs.

Figure 4-1 Mail Enclosure (Front)

STEVEN JENKINS, Ph.D.
PSYCHOLOGIST
1 North Main Street
Providence, Rhode Island 02853

(401) 123-4567

BASIS FOR PSYCHOLOGICAL REFERRAL

CHILD

Presenting Problems

1. Prolonged poor school performance, particularly if onset was sudden
2. Nightmares for over 3 weeks
3. Hyperkinetic reaction—organic or functional**
4. Poor relations with peers
5. Unable to be "managed" by parents**
6. Phobic reactions (including school phobia)

**Likelihood of family therapy indicated.

ADOLESCENT

Presenting Problems

1. Immediate referral if suicide is alluded to
2. Poor school performance with sudden onset
3. Withdrawing reactions
4. Where drug or alcohol is involved
5. Sexual difficulties, including pregnancy
6. Explosive personality or over-aggressive reactions

As with any form of announcement, attention must be paid to ethical considerations. The letter should be sent only once and only to referral sources, not to potential patients.

DIRECT CONTACT

At some point personal contact should be made with potential referral sources. Since these meetings take from 30 to 60 minutes plus travel time, potential referral sources should be carefully selected. A practitioner, for example, interested in the geriatric population will develop different referral sources than a practitioner interested in a pediatric population. Figure 4-2 provides suggested referral contacts for five major therapeutic groups.

To some degree each category of referral source should be handled differently. Each has particular interests, training and obligations, and unless the therapist is sensitive to these, communication may be thwarted.

Figure 4-1 Mail Enclosure (Reverse)

STEVEN JENKINS, Ph.D.
PSYCHOLOGIST
1 North Main Street
Providence, Rhode Island 02853
——
(401) 123-4567

REFERRAL PROCEDURE

CHILDREN

1. Simply have the patient's parent or guardian call the above number.
2. Dr. Jenkins will personally arrange an appointment for your patient.

ADOLESCENTS

1. Depending upon your discretion, either the patient or his parents may call for an appointment.
2. Adolescents who call on their own for an appointment will be seen by Dr. Jenkins without their parents for the first interview. Parent involvement will be discussed at that time.

Figure 4-2

REFERRAL SOURCES FOR STAGES OF

DEVELOPMENT

Children
    Pediatricians
    Pediatric Neurologists
    Family and general medical practitioners
    Lawyers (for custody and divorce)
    Family Court
    School Departments
    Child Welfare Department
    Military Medical installations
    Other Mental Health Service organizations

Adult
    Family and general medical practitioners
    Gynecologists, Obstetricians, Urologists (Sexual
    problems)
    Neurologist, Internist, Orthopedic Surgeon (Psy-
    chosomatic Disorders and Pain)
    Department of Labor (Vocational Rehabilitation)
    Clergy
    Other Mental Health Services Organizations

Adolescents
    Physicians
    Lawyers
    Family Court
    Police Department (Juvenile Division)
    School Departments
    Military Medical Installations

Geriatric
    Physicians
    Clergy
    Nursing Homes
    Senior Citizen Organizations

Physicians

Physicians are the main source of referrals to mental health practitioners. They are often looked to by their patients for advice on a multitude of problems, perhaps because they are still perceived as parent figures.

For the beginning practitioner, more recently established physicians are usually easier to cultivate than seasoned physicians whose referral patterns are probably well established. And, unfortunately, doctors trained in the 1940's and 1950's are of a generation that has serious misgivings about mental health practitioners. Younger physicians have been exposed to the concept of the intimate link between physical and mental health.

Hospital Staff. The fastest way to develop physician contacts is to join a hospital staff. While this type of affiliation is traditionally much easier for a psychiatrist to accomplish than a psychologist or social worker, there is a recent trend toward incorporating these clinicians in some way into the hospital staff. While a psychiatrist may be able to enjoy full staff privileges, psychologists or social workers may find themselves relegated to roles of less status.

The typical hospital staff hierarchy is as follows:

Active medical staff, with full voting privileges regarding hospital policy is usually composed primarily of physicians and dentists who have passed a probationary period;

Associate medical staff have all the qualifications and most of the privileges of the Active Staff but is comprised of new members who usually remain at this probationary status for one to three years.

Affiliate Staff, Consulting Staff or *Courtesy Staff* are honorary designations with limited privileges that seldom include admitting or voting. This status might entail such obligations as attending staff and departmental meetings and performing or being available to perform specific services at the hospital at certain times.

Regardless of the level of hospital affiliation, some

benefits will accrue to the mental health practitioner. Even if a psychologist or a social worker does not enjoy full privileges and responsibilities, staff meetings and other hospital functions, including social ones help him become known to the medical staff. Certainly, questions regarding the clinician's credentials are quickly laid to rest, since credential review is necessary to become a staff member in any capacity.

Applying for Membership. The therapist's first step toward joining a hospital staff is writing a brief letter to the administrator or medical director indicating his desire for affiliation. The response to that letter will include some explanation of the hospital staff and structure and application procedure and materials. Usually, the application is first given to a specific department for scrutiny. This might be a department of psychiatry, psychology or social services, depending on the size and orientation of the hospital. The application may then go to a credentials committee, an executive committee and finally to a full staff meeting for a vote. Usually, there will be an interview prior to the final vote.

If the hospital is departmentalized—and most hospitals are—each department defines to some degree its areas of responsibility and expectations of its members. All hospital staff are usually assigned to one of these departments. However, unless the practitioner wishes to take an active role, such as providing emergency room consultation or some other concrete service, departmental assignment will not be critical.

Hospital affiliation is of value to a therapist only if it allows other physicians to become acquainted with his skills. Attendance at meetings therefore, is a critical form of exposure. Also, some consideration should be given to conducting a hospital workshop or continuing education program in order to familiarize others with one's areas of interest and expertise. Typical mental health practitioner programs deal with managing patient stress, assessment of psychological correleates in organic disease, clinical hypnosis, and other topics.

Initial Contact. The following dialogue typifies an initial contact between an experienced practitioner and a referral source.

Receptionist: Dr. Gibbs' office.

Doctor Young: Hello, this is Dr. Young calling for Dr. Gibbs . . . Is he available?

Receptionist: He's just finishing up with a patient. I'll tell him that you're calling. Would you hold the line for a second?

Dr. Young: Of course. (A 90-second delay.)

Dr. Gibbs: Jerry Gibbs here.

Dr. Young: Hi, Jerry. This is Bob Young. I'm a psychiatrist and I just opened an office on Phillips Street. I'd like to get together with you and let you know what services I'll be providing. . . . I don't know what your schedule is like, but would a lunchtime meeting be convenient for you?

Dr. Gibbs: Well, let me take a look at my schedule. Things have really been hopping around here, and I don't think I'm going to be able to get away until the end of the week. . . . How about lunch on Friday?

Dr. Young: That sounds good to me. Do you have a particular place in mind?

Dr. Gibbs: Well, the Red Coach Inn has pretty good lunches.

Dr. Young: Fine. Is noon a good time for you?

Dr. Gibbs: That's fine. I might be just a couple of minutes late. As a matter of fact, why don't you call my receptionist on Thursday and have her remind me about lunch?

Dr. Young: Just fine. I'm looking forward to seeing you.

In this conversation, Dr. Young immediately identifies himself, indicates his desire to talk with Dr. Gibbs, permits the receptionist some leeway by asking if Dr. Gibbs is available. With this strategy, Dr. Young is likely to be connected. While the 90-second wait might seem very long, it may have been necessary if Dr. Gibbs was trying to complete a procedure. It would be unfortunate if Dr. Young perceived the wait as Dr. Gibbs' rudeness. Unless one is certain he has been disconnected or the call has been forgotten, it is best to wait up to 4 or 5 minutes before redialing.

Because Dr. Gibbs provided it, protocol permitted Dr.

Young to use Dr. Gibbs' first name. Also, Dr. Young extended the same courtesy. Some practitioners, however, prefer being addressed by their title.

Luncheon Meeting. Luncheon meetings tend to be more relaxed and more successful than other types of meetings in establishing feelings of trust. Although a certain amount of data will be exchanged, the meeting is primarily an opportunity for two people to know each other and determine whether or not a beneficial professional relationship can develop. The referral source will be consciously or unconsciously trying to determine how his patients might respond to the therapist. At the same time, the therapist will find out something about the referral source's knowledge of and attitude toward therapy and the possible use he might make of such services.

The tone of the meeting and the material covered will vary according to the setting and the individuals. However, some time during the course of the meeting, the therapist should provide the referral source with information about his training, orientation and preferred clientele. Also, the therapist should learn how much feedback the referral source requires concerning his patients. Most important, some format for referrals should be established. Some doctors like to have business cards of practitioners to whom they refer patients. The therapist can indicate that he will send the doctor a few cards, thus affording himself the opportunity of establishing another contact. In any event, the therapist should not be embarrassed about handing out a card.

Other Meeting Places. Occasionally, a physician may ask to meet the therapist in his office or at a hospital cafeteria. These meetings should be handled somewhat differently. The hospital cafeteria is an uncomfortable meeting place. Conversation is awkward in a cafeteria line; tables must often be shared with strangers; there may be interruptions from colleagues; the constant drone of the hospital public address system is distracting. If the meeting must be at the hospital, the therapist should ask if a conference room might be acquired.

Meeting in the doctor's office may be a matter of convenience or may reflect defensiveness on the part of the physician. Such meetings are likely to be restrained. If the doctor's schedule is full, the therapist may be regarded as intruding on his earning ability and may be mentally grouped with drug salesmen. Such meetings should be brief and introductory, allowing the therapist to learn something about the physician's office demeanor. If the physician remains behind his desk and the therapist in front, there may be a strong press to play out well-established doctor-patient roles. This situation is not terribly conducive for establishing a referral relationship but would be indicative of the way the physician feels comfortable operating on initial contact.

Being Direct. There is no harm in letting someone know that one's purpose in meeting with him is to receive referrals. When one physician asked why a therapist wanted to meet him, the therapist, taken aback slightly, said, "So that you can refer patients to me." To his surprise, the physician agreed to meet, and eventually became a very reliable referral source.

Schools

It is customary to have meetings with school personnel at the school. Many school officials feel that employees are not working unless they are in school. Employees are often concerned that being seen out of school will be construed as lack of performance by a member of the community. The therapist might reciprocate in the future by inviting the referral source to meet with him in his office, a more businesslike setting than a local restaurant. Meeting in the school cafeteria is definitely not recommended.

Contacting School Personnel. It is helpful to respect hierarchy and regulations of the school. Unless the practitioner already knows a referral source there, his first contact should be with the school superintendent.

In the initial phone conversation, the therapist should identify himself and his profession, indicate that he has opened an office nearby, and request a meeting. The superintendent may provide the name of someone with whom he feels it more appropriate for the therapist to meet, for example, the director of pupil personnel services or the director of special education.

From this point, contact will probably be with personnel indicated by the superintendent. Although it is rare for a superintendent to be involved in referring students, protocol requires that he be contacted prior to contacting any other staff. In the same regard, the school principal should be contacted before other staff in his building are contacted.

Unless he has been instructed otherwise, the therapist should *always* check in at the school office when making a visit. At some schools he will be expected to sign in and out. During the initial visit, it is both polite and constructive to ask for a tour of the building. School personnel usually take pride in their building and will feel the therapist is more familiar with their situation if they show him around.

It will be helpful if the therapist has some understanding of school schedules, reading programs, types of textbooks, reasonable class size, etc. Such knowledge will increase his credibility with the school.

Military Bases. A nearby military installation can be a major referral source. Military chaplains frequently look for assistance in working with difficult pastoral counseling cases, and pediatricians and other specialists at the base hospital may also need support. The names of the head chaplain, chief of pediatrics, and other staff can be obtained from the switchboard.

Other Sources are correctional facilities, churches, homes for the aged, self help groups (such as Parents without Partners or Parents Anonymous), police departments, departments of vocational rehabilitation, social welfare and child protection agencies, adoption agencies, and the court system. Each agency or system will have its own idiocyncracies about which the therapist will quickly learn. Continual contact over long periods frequently result in referrals. Other sources of referrals may include friends, other therapists and civic organizations such as the Lions Club or Masons, but these are usually not as productive as those mentioned above.

Other Strategies

Free Lectures. Delivering lectures to civic and special-interest groups often results in referrals. Sometimes mental health associations have a list of speakers which they make available upon request. One psychiatrist who volunteered to lecture through several organizations when he started practice, eventually gave as many as two free talks a week. Within a year he not only had a waiting list of patients but became a major referral source himself. Few therapists are so dynamic, but time volunteered in presenting topical programs is well rewarded.

Workshops for a Fee. It is ideal to be able to give a talk or workshop for a fee. This not only creates exposure but helps supplement income. The greatest market for such workshops are schools. Other sources may include industry, nursing homes and special interest groups.

A news release about a talk or workshop should be submitted to the local paper. The release should include information about the program and the therapist's role in it. Such visibility may stimulate interest for other programs and have a cumulative effect on potential referrals. Chapter Nine provides more details about this strategy.

5

RECORD KEEPING

Hank, a luncheonette owner, has, through careful management and hard work been able to support his family and send one of his children to college. He has two employees: a dishwasher and a waitress who comes in during the rush time. He has a good accountant and lawyer, keeps careful books, and can give an accurate picture of his financial condition at any time. Further down the street, Dr. Harvey Stone, a respected psychotherapist who has been in practice for three years, may gross $45,000 this year but isn't sure because his books are not very accurate. When Dr. Stone began his practice on a part-time basis of three to four hours a week, he kept most of his financial records in a spiral stenographic note book. Unfortunately, he has never updated his record keeping.

There is more fact than fiction in the above story. Many small businessmen with moderate incomes employ more sophisticated financial management techniques than therapists who earn much more money. In addition to the risk of failing to survive an IRS audit, poor records may hide errors in the therapist's favor. (Patients and insurance companies will find those errors that are in *their* favor.) This chapter deals with establishing office procedures that insure efficient record keeping.

THE APPOINTMENT BOOK

A matter as simple as the style of an appointment book can affect one's income. If the layout of the book is confusing, appointment times may be accidentally left unfilled. For an individual practice, a book showing the entire week on a page large enough to accommodate each hourly appointment is recommended. Books that show the entire month on a page usually cannot accommodate twelve appointment hours for each day. Books with one day per page tend to be bulky and scheduling weekly appointments involves flipping through a series of pages. Group practice requires a master appointment book in which one page is used for each day, with separate columns or page sections designated for different therapists.

There are some common and costly errors to be avoided. Unless canceled appointments are noted *at the time of cancellation*, the therapist may forget and have an unwanted free hour. Also, some therapists are remiss in entering new appointments or re-entering weekly appointments. This can result in double scheduling or missing appointments. Such an oversight can lead to loss of income and also to the loss of a patient.

SETTING UP BOOKS

The Checking Account

The first financial rule in setting up any business is to separate personal from business finances by opening a commercial checking account in the name of the business. If the practice is incorporated, the therapist has no choice: business expenses cannot be paid from his personal account. All receipts from patients, either cash or check, should be deposited into the business account. The therapist's salary (or draw) and all other business expenses should be paid by check from this account. If those two rules are followed, the check ledger, deposit slips, and canceled checks will function as an important financial record of the practice and will be helpful in the event of an IRS audit.

It is critical that the account be balanced promptly each month so that errors are not compounded. Checks should never be written to cash except for the therapist's own salary or draw which can then be deposited in his personal account. Checks should be kept for at least three years, which is the statute of limitations for tax audit not involving fraud (there is no limitation for fraud).

Patient Receipts

There are three records of patients' receipts: the daily log indicates who was seen, the fee charged and the fee paid; the patient's personal ledger card lists in chronological order all his financial transactions; the receipt for each transaction given to the patient.

For any practice of over 6 hours a week, a preprinted receipt/ledger system is recommended. The system, which costs about $170 with forms for 1500 transactions, includes ledger cards for each patient printed with the therapist's name and address. Figure 5-1 shows the type of ledger card frequently provided in a preprinted system. The card is divided into columns for date, patient's name, services rendered, fee, credits and balance. It is possible to have codes printed in the bottom portion of the card which can be used to simplify billing. The card can be easily photocopied, folded and mailed in a windowed envelope also to simplify billing.

Day sheets and transaction slips, Figure 5-2, are also included in the system. The day sheet provides for a chrono-

Figure 5-1

STATEMENT

ALLEN G. SHEFFIELD, ACSW
19 SALINA STREET
RIVERVIEW, MASS. 12345

TELEPHONE
617–921–3111

CHARGES OR
PAYMENTS MADE
AFTER LAST DATE
SHOWN WILL APPEAR
ON YOUR NEXT
STATEMENT

BALANCE
FORWARD

DATE - FAMILY MEMBER	DESCRIPTION	TOTAL FEE	CREDITS		BALANCE
			PAYMENTS	ADJ.	

SAFEGUARD BUSINESS SYSTEMS Form No. LS-M-11

PLEASE PAY LAST AMOUNT IN BALANCE COLUMN —⬏

DI—Diagnostic Interview
IT—Individual Therapy
GT—Group Therapy
FT—Family Therapy
PT—Psychological Testing
FKA—Failure To Keep
    Appointment

C—Consultation
SC—School Consultation
HC—Hospital Consultation
ROA—Received on Account

eprinted by permission of Safeguard Business Systems, Inc.
rt Washington Industrial Park
rt Washington, Pa. 19034

Figure 5-2

Transaction Slip

PATIENT'S NAME

Please present this slip to receptionist before leaving office

PREVIOUS BALANCE

DI—Diagnostic Interview...............
IT—Individual Therapy ....
GT—Group Therapy ....
FT—Family Therapy ....
PT—Psychological Testing ....
FKA—Failure To Keep Appointment
C—Consultation ....
SC—School Consultation ....
HC—Hospital Consultation...............
ROA—Received on Account ....

TOTAL

1546 ___ DAYS ___ WKS ___ MO.

DATE | FAMILY MEMBER | DESCRIPTION | TOTAL FEE | PAYMENT | ADJ. | BALANCE
CREDITS

This is your RECEIPT for this amount
This is a STATEMENT of your account to date

ALLEN G. SHEFFIELD, ACSW

19 SALINA STREET
RIVERVIEW, MASS. 12345

TELEPHONE:
617-921-3111

DI—Diagnostic Interview
IT—Individual Therapy
GT—Group Therapy
FT—Family Therapy
PT—Psychological Testing

FKA—Failure To Keep Appointment
C—Consultation
SC—School Consultation
HC—Hospital Consultation
ROA—Received on Account

Appointments Not Cancelled At Least 24 Hours In Advance Are Charged At Full Rate.

Thank You

YOUR NEXT APPOINTMENT WILL BE

PATIENT NAME | DATE | DAY | TIME

1546

Reprinted by permission of Safeguard Business Systems, Inc.
Fort Washington Industrial Park
Fort Washington, Pa. 19034

logical account of all transactions and is designed so that all transactions can be "proved" or balanced. It also provides for day-to-day and month-to-month review of accounts receivable (money owed). These items are designed to be used in a special ledger which permits all three transactions to be recorded simultaneously.

Such a system is, in the final analysis, not very costly. Printed ledger cards which are photocopied and placed in windowed envelopes save billing time and expense. The system also facilitates day to day assessment of accounts receivable. Loss of control over these accounts can be a serious problem for practitioners.

Purchase of a commercial ledger system is not absolutely necessary and would be an extravagance for a practitioner with only two to five patients a week. However, certain aspects of the system should be adhered to even by the therapist with only one patient a month. The clinician should have a ledger card as previously described for every patient. Stationery and business supply stores carry ruled or lined cards that can easily be used for this purpose. Index cards can also be used. The cards should be filed in a small metal box or tray, with alphabetic dividers for easy reference. Without ledger cards, the difficulty in reconstructing a patient's account may be insurmountable. A record kept on an index card can be readily transferred to billing stationery.

A simple ledger book or bookkeeping paper housed in a binder can substitute for a day or week sheet. Figure 5-3 pictures one such system. It is important that every transaction entered include the patient's name, the date, type of transaction and fee, amount paid, and the current and previous balance. The previous balance can be obtained from the patient's account card. Mr. Smith, in Figure 5-3, had no previous balance, was seen one hour, and charged $40 which he paid. His current balance, therefore, is zero. Mrs. Jones owed $80, was seen half an hour, charged $20 which she did not pay, and her current balance is $100. Mr. Brown,who was not seen, mailed in a check for $110. Since his previous balance was $200, his current balance is $90. In adding up the columns, one sees that $60 was charged that day (column A), $150 paid (column B), $190 still owed (column D) by patients who previously owed $280 (column E). The following formula proves the account:

$$Column\ (E+A)-B-C=Column\ D.$$

$$(280+60)-150-0=190$$

Adjustments (column C) are used when the full fee is not expected or obtainable. An adjustment is a way of lowering a fee or writing off a bad debt. If, for example, an insurance company pays a portion of a bill for someone who cannot pay the difference, entering that difference as an adjustment removes the patient from the accounts receivable.

The receipt or transaction slip consists of one or two parts. Since it contains the information recorded in the patient's account ledger, it can be used by him for his tax records or for submitting an insurance claim. Two-part transaction slips contain small coupons which can be used by the therapist and his receptionist. They show the previous balance (for the therapist's information) and current charges (for the receptionist's information). While helpful in group practices, these coupons are usually superfluous in individual practice.

About Accounts Receivable

Deciding what number of accounts receivable is acceptable is like evaluating the track record of a thoracic surgeon. If all his patients die in surgery, the surgeon might be suspected of malpractice. If all his patients live, one might suspect that he is operating on people who are not seriously ill. So it goes with accounts receivable. If a practitioner never collects a penny, he is mismanaging his practice clinically and financially. On the other hand, a practitioner who collects 100% of his fees might be restricting his practice to an afflu-

Figure 5-3
Day Sheet

DATE / FAMILY MEMBER	DESCRIPTION	A TOTAL FEE	B PAY-MENTS	C ADJ.	D CURRENT BALANCE	√	E PREVIOUS BALANCE	NAME	TRANS-ACTION NO.
								Carry forward from today's totals - only if more than one page is used today →	
1-6	Individual Therapy (1 hour)	40 —	40 —		—			Mrs. Smith	1
1-7	" (½ hr.)	20 —			100 —		80 —	Mrs. Jones	2
1-7	ROA		110 —		90 —		200 —	Mr. Brown	3
									4
									5
									6
									7
									8
									9
									10
TOTALS		A 60 —	B 150 —	C	D 190 —		E 280 —	Carry forward to top of next page, only if more than one page is used today. →	
THIS PAGE OR TODAY'S TOTAL →					→ PREV. DAY MONTH-TO-DATE TOTAL				
					→ MONTH-TO-DATE TOTAL				

PAGE PROOF OF POSTING
COL. E + A - B - C = COL. D

DAY SHEET
RECORD OF CHARGES AND RECEIPTS
SAFEGUARD BUSINESS SYSTEMS, INC. 1976

Safeguard
Form No. OVJ - M11

Provided through courtesy of Safeguard Business Systems, Inc.

65

ent and fiscally responsible population. Most accountants agree that over a year's time outstanding accounts receivable should be between 10% and 20% of fees charged.

According to collection agencies, the older a receivable account, the less likelihood of it being collected. Generally, receivable accounts older than 90 days are collected less than 40% of the time. The following formula can be used to calculate the current total of accounts receivable (A/R).

(Day's charges − day's payments) − day's adjustments = day's A/R

Day's A/R + prior total A/R to date = current total A/R

To prove A/R, add all column A (fees charged) to date and subtract from that all columns B & C (credits). That number should equal the total A/R.

To calculate the percentage of accounts receivable, divide the total A/R by the total of column A to date.

In order to facilitate the above calculations, it is important to keep cumulative totals of all the columns by the day or week. This is an excellent method of presentation for an IRS audit. Comparing the running A/R balance to the credit and charge columns eliminates the possibility of errors or unintentional misappropriations. One can keep track of earnings by running a cumulative total of credits. Earnings which have been previously taxed (such as a university salary) should not be entered here. A separate record is kept of such income in the check register or in a special ledger book.

Expense Ledger

A double entry expense ledger permits the practitioner to prove his books and determine how much money is being spent for various needs. The ledger, as seen in Figure 5-4, consists of a series of columns, each representing a different category of expenditure. A 12-column ledger should be sufficient for most practices. It is imperative that every expenditure, whether paid by check or currency, is entered as soon as possible after it is made. Since most columns represent legitimate business expenses, an up-to-date accurate expense ledger greatly facilitates tax calculations.

Posting the Expense Ledger. Figure 5-4 shows the way in which the expense ledger should be posted: the date of the transaction in column A; the check number in column B; the check recipient in column D; the amount of the check in column E and in any special category designated in section F. A payroll column may be added for corporations or practices with employees. Column C is used for noting cash transactions in lieu of a petty cash fund which can be cumbersome and difficult to record. Whenever cash is spent, a receipt should be kept and numbered, and that number entered in column C. The receipts for the month can be stored in an envelope for the month, with current month's envelope taped to the inside of the back binder of the ledger. These will prove an indispensable aid at audit time.

The ten common expense categories used in private practice are shown in Figure 5-4. The number and labels of the columns can be changed to suit each practice.

Column 1: Consultative Services. This includes a payment for contracted secretarial, typing, or cleaning services and any other labor for which withholding taxes have not been deducted. The therapist's own wage is never entered in this category.

Column 2: Supplies, Postage. Items that are quickly used up or consumed are listed here. These include stamps, UPS charges, stationary, pencils, test answer sheets, coffee, etc.

Column 3: Rented Services. Answering service expenses should be recorded here and service contracts for equipment such as a typewriter or airconditioner. Rental of such equipment as a photocopy machine, postage meter, typewriter, dictating equipment or answering machine can also be included.

Column 4: Rent. If a site is rented for business only the full amount can be recorded here. If the office is in one's

Figure 5-4
Expense Ledger

A Date	B Check No.	C Receipt No.	D Payee	E Total	F 1 Outside Office Help	2 Supplies Postage Etc.	3 Rental Services	4 Rent	5 Utilities	6 Entertainment & Adv.	7 Misc.	8	9 Equipment	10 Non-deduct.
197—														
1-1	101		A. Smith	150 —				150 —						
1-2	102		Book Club	25 —		25 —								
1-3	103		U.S. Postmaster stamps	10 —		10 —								
1-8	Cash	1	Red Coach Inn	27 80						27 80				
1-9	104		Sue White typist	85 —	85 —									
1-10	105		Answering Service	30 —			30 —							
1-11	106		Electric Co.	18 —					18 —					
1-11	Cash	2	Acme Market	2 49										2 49
1-16	107		Hank's Furniture chair	153 —									153 —	
1-17	108		Quick Printing Co.	32 —		32 —								

rented home, only a percentage of the rent should be entered.* That percentage is based on the following formula:

$$\frac{\text{sq. feet of office area}}{\text{total sq. feet of all usable living area}} \times \text{Rent} = \text{Office Rent.}$$

If, for example, a house is 1000 square feet and one 200 square foot room is used as an office, 20% of the rent may be considered a business expense. If the monthly rent is $350, $70 should be entered in column 4, although the full $350 will be paid from the personal checking account.

Recent tax reforms prohibit declaring any space not used solely for business.

If one owns a building one may not declare rent expense. However, an accountant should be consulted for information about depreciation deduction.

Column 5: Utilities. These include gas, electricity, water, telephone, garbage and fire service. If the practice is located in one's home the same proportion should be deducted as would be for rent. That percentage also applies to the telephone base charge, but, toll calls and message units must be itemized as in column 4. Expenses are paid from one's personal account, but the business proportion recorded in column 5.

Column 6: Entertainment and Advertising. Most practitioners feel they do not advertise. However, expenses that fall into this category include mail announcements, business cards, signs, newspaper announcements, and workshop handouts. Gifts to referral sources come under this category. Entertainment includes business lunches, parties and other events detailed in Chapter 4. A separate record of entertainment expenses should include location, persons attending and the purpose of the event.

Column 7: Miscellaneous. This category encompasses

*The IRS has progressively restricted deductions of this type, particularly if one has an office outside the home.

such occasional expenses as attorney, accountant, and other professional fees; dues; workshops and other education expenses; out-of-town travel related to the practice; minor fees and repairs; interest on loans (repayment of principal is posted in column 10). If one miscellaneous item gains in importance or frequency, it can be given a heading in column 8.

Column 8: This can be used for any other category important to the practice. For example, salaries in practices where employees are involved.

Column 9: Equipment. Large items that have a useful life of over one year and can be considered for tax credits or depreciation allowance are recorded here. These include furniture, fixtures, test kits (Rorschach and WAIS, for example, but not expendable material such as answer sheets) and biofeedback instruments.

Column 10: Nondeductible Miscellaneous. These include the therapist's draw, fines and penalties, and repayments of loan principal (interest is entered in column 7).

Proving the Ledger. When the columns are totaled at the end of the month, the total of column E should equal the total of all the columns in section F. At the end of the year, the cumulative totals for all the columns are the basis for tax deductions (except Column 10).

Automobile Expenses. Automobile expenses can be handled in one of two ways. One method is to record business mileage and take the standard mileage allowance provided by the IRS. In that case, auto expenses are not entered in the expense ledger. The alternative method involves recording all automobile expenses such as gas, oil, tune ups, etc. in a separate column for example, column 8 in the ledger. An accountant can best advise about which method to use. Unless a luxury car has been purchased for the practice, most accountants advise declaring mileage rather than expenses when business travel exceeds 4500 miles a year.

Adequate record keeping is necessary whichever system is used. Mileage can be recorded in an inexpensive booklet intended for this purpose and kept in the glove compartment of the car. The beginning and ending odometer reading of each trip is recorded. The tax laws regarding business mileage are under revision. Currently, travel from home to business is considered a commuting expense and is non-deductible. However, mileage *between* offices, from the office to a consultation, or from home to a workshop is deductible. Also, all tolls paid for business travel are deductible.

Cash vs. Accrual Accounting

In accrual accounting, accounts receivable are recorded as if the money had been already received. That is if a patient is seen and charged $40, the $40 is recorded as income whether or not it is paid. This system, used most frequently by companies dealing in merchandising and inventory, permits a tax deduction for bad debts.

In cash accounting, money is recorded as income only when it is received. In this system, bad debts may not be considered a tax deduction. In private practice, there is little advantage in using the accrual system. It is cumbersome and more difficult than the cash system to manage for private practitioners.

6 PRIVATE PRACTICE AS A BUSINESS

In this chapter, corporations, taxes, fees and other aspects of business as it applies to a practice will be discussed.

FEES

Setting Fees

There is no iron clad rule for setting fees. Most Professional Standard Review Organizations (PSRO) and insurance companies consider a fee to be usual and customary if it is within the 90th percentile of fees charged by all practitioners in the same field and geographic region. It is recommended that most beginners set their fees fairly close to the 90th percentile. Novices are sometimes apologetic about setting fees, at the 90th percentile but most seasoned practitioners find that such fees do not discourage patients from seeking their services. One danger in setting fees too low is that when the therapist finds he must raise his fee, insurance companies may provide reimbursement based on the old fee. A therapist can make exceptions occasionally and adjust a single fee downward without effecting his profile.

A therapist can conduct his own survey of fees by calling several practitioners in his area. At the time of this book's publication, according to *Psychotherapy Finances* (February, 1978), the median hourly fee charged by therapists throughout the country was $40, with $45 representing the 90th percentile. However, fees varied according to discipline and geographic area.

Raising Fees

As a rule, it is unwise to raise fees of existing patients. It causes resentment and might be regarded as a breach of contract. If it is absolutely necessary to raise all patients' fees, reasonable advance notice should be given.

Collection of Fees

There is a tremendous advantage in having patients pay after each session. It saves billing costs, provides the therapist with immediate funds, and, most important, reduces the possibility of bad debts. The therapist's attitude about immediate payment can affect patient response. If he is at ease and matter of fact in explaining to new patients his preference for that procedure, they are more likely to conform to it.

However, therapists occasionally have patients who terminate owing money and with no intention of paying the debt. Such patients sometimes give clues beforehand that they are likely not to pay. Frequently, clients who claim financial prowess but expect to be billed for services become delinquent in payment. If this problem comes up while the client is still in therapy, it is, of course, appropriate to discuss its clinical aspects. In the meantime, however, the client should be expected to bring his account up to date and pay weekly.

Certain types of cases or consultations are prone to payment problems. These include hospital evaluations of any sort, particularly orthopedic or other consultations in which the physician believes there may be psychological reasons for pain. Such patients sometimes resent their physicians for suggesting that the pain is psychological. The referrals are often a result of the physician's frustration and bewilderment. The mental health practitioner then suffers from the patient's hostility by not being paid.

Practitioners handle these cases in different ways, depending on the extent of insurance benefits. Unless the therapist plans to do volunteer work, he should educate the referring physician about the necessary financial arrangements for hospital consultations. The therapist should try to determine in advance whether the patient is insured for his services. If he is, the therapist should secure from the hospital business office a form by which the patient authorizes the insurance company to pay the therapist directly. Unless he does this, the patient might not forward the reimbursement to the therapist. Some practitioners require that the patient or a family member sign a form agreeing to pay the consultation fee and explain that such fees may not be covered by hospitalization insurance. If a therapist uses this method, he should have a nurse or the referring physician ask the patient to fill out the form so that the wary patient does not see the therapist as a money grabber. The form does not insure payment, but those who use it claim that it reduces misunderstandings.

Family therapy might also present collection problems, particularly if financial stress is presented as a principal problem. The family should be helped to understand that payment must be made after each session, even if the person who normally pays it is not present.

Court referral might also be problematic. Patients sometimes unconsciously resent the referral and may even consciously feel the judge should pay for the visits. In cases where evaluations are being performed for custody, liability or criminal court cases, the therapist should make it a policy to collect after each visit or at least before his report is submitted. To avoid problems with the referring lawyer, the therapist should send a letter outlining his fees for evaluations and court appearances. He may ask either that the evaluation be paid for in advance or that the lawyer guarantee payment upon submission of the report.

A credit bureau will confirm that the longer a bill goes uncollected, the less likelihood there is of payment ever being received. Even if payment is eventually made, the therapist has lost the use of those funds during the period the bill was outstanding. Unless he is prepared to write off debts, the therapist should take certain steps to insure payment. First, he should make an effort to send bills out promptly. If he is carefree in billing patients, they may respond similarly. If he does not receive a response within 30 days, another copy of the bill marked "Second Notice" should be sent out. If another 30 days goes by without payment, the therapist has reason to suspect that the bill will be difficult to collect. At this point he has two choices.

He can call the patient and remind him that payment is more than 60 days late. In the conversation he should try to determine the nature of the patient's reluctance to pay. He should also try to get a specific commitment concerning payment. If the patient says, "I'll send you a check right away," the therapist should ask, "By what date?" and "For how much will the check be?" His reply should be repeated so that both therapist and patient understand the commitment.

Instead of calling, the therapist can write on a copy of the bill, "Bill must be paid within 15 days" (the due date should be noted on the bill). Many patients respond to this type of non-threatening assertion. If there is no reply, the following letter may be sent to the client:

Would you please call the office to indicate why your account should not be turned over for collection by (give a date 15 days in advance).

If there is still no reply, after all the notices have been sent, 4 choices remain.

1) The account can be referred to a collection attorney.
2) The account can be referred to a collection agency.
3) The therapist can take the case to small claims court himself.
4) The therapist can drop the matter.

If the bill is less than $15, the last option is advised. If the amount is greater than that, any of the three other options are viable. There are a few things to consider before choosing the first or second option. Most attorneys and virtually all collection agencies work on a commission basis and receive a fee only if they succeed in collecting the account. The average fee is a third of the amount collected. If the case comes to court, the therapist may have to pay a filing fee or a process server's fee. In either case, the charges are not likely to exceed $20. The attorney or agency selected should be accustomed to working for professionals (particularly medical) who provide services rather than commodities and should be ethical. An overzealous or aggressive attorney who immediately threatens to take a lien on the client's home or to garnishee his wages reflects poorly on the therapist professionally.

Turning an account over for collection does not guarantee payment. The client may be unresponsive to the collection agency's or attorney's demands. At some point, the therapist may have to decide whether or not to take legal action. Most attorneys are not interested in handling a law suit unless at least several hundred dollars are involved.

Some practitioners take cases to small claims court rather than go to a collection agency or attorney. Small claims courts hear cases involving amounts less than $500 or $600, depending upon the laws of the state. The proceedings are simple enough so that an attorney is not needed. The two parties present their sides to a judge who renders a decision, either at the time of the hearing or shortly thereafter. Most small claims hearings take place within 30 days after the initial filing, which in some cases must take place in the county seat of the defendant. The cost of filing the petition in the County Clerk's office is usually only a few dollars.

The advantages of filing in small claims court are that the case can be resolved quickly and there are no attorney or agency fees involved. The disadvantage is the time that must be spent filing and participating in the proceedings. Also, the complainant must waive his right to appeal the judge's decision.

The obvious lesson here is to avoid situations which result in accumulation of accounts receivable much beyond 30 days. However, some uncollectable accounts are normal. After all, the only way to avoid this situation completely is to have people pay in advance. Such distrust would do little to promote a practice.

In a very few cases, nonpayment reflects a legitimate misunderstanding or anger on the part of the patient. If the therapist feels that there is a misunderstanding, he may choose to telephone the client and try to resolve it. If the client is very angry, the therapist should keep in mind that legal action on his part might result in the client retaliating by suing for malpractice. Although, as mentioned in Chapter 10, only a small number of malpractice suits against mental health practitioners have been successful, such a suit may involve a considerable expenditure of time and energy. This risk should be weighed against any possible financial benefit.

ACCOUNTS PAYABLE

The other side of accounts receivable is accounts payable, which include such expenses as telephone, rent, answering service and legal fees. Bi-monthly payments are frequent enough to keep current on the most urgent bills and take advantage of nominal discounts for prompt payment offered by some companies. Bi-monthly payments also lend more stability to cash flow, that is, the balance of money received and money paid out.

Borrowing Money

At various times in his career, the private practitioner may need to borrow money. There is no shame in this, nor is it a sign that he is in dire financial straits. One obvious reason for borrowing is to make a large purchase of property or equipment. There are other circumstances in which loans are in order. If for example, a substantial portion of a therapist's patients are covered by CHAMPUS, health insurance for military dependents, and administration changes delay checks by 6 to 8 weeks, the therapist will not be financially fluid. In this circumstance many practitioners might borrow a low interest 30-90 day discount note.

Some banks also offer a "personal line of credit." The interest on this is higher than on a discount note, but it is a convenient method of borrowing. After the application is approved, any amount up to the agreed upon limit can be borrowed. Interest is charged only for the time the money is used, with minimum payment required each month, usually 10%–50% of the principal depending on its size.

It is necessary to fill out an application for a loan or, in the case of a note, a financial statement. A loan officer can assist with the financial statement. In borrowing money one should remember that the bank is in business to make money by lending it. One need not feel ashamed of borrowing or grateful for being allowed to borrow. It is worthwhile shopping around for the lowest interest rates. There is no harm in asking for a rate reduction of half a point. It is also important to borrow enough money. There is nothing more frustrating than borrowing $2500 only to find out later that one really needed $3000.

SETTING UP A BUSINESS STRUCTURE

Sole Proprietorships

A sole proprietorship is the simplest and most common form of practice. It is a term used to describe an unincorporated business owned by one individual. From a business and tax standpoint, no legal arrangements are necessary to open a practice in sole proprietorship unless the practice is given a name other than the practitioner's, such as "Therapy Associates" or "South County Psychiatric Service." In that case, it is necessary to file a Trade Name Certificate with the town or city clerk. The certificate simply states that Dr. Joseph Smith will be doing business as "Therapy Associates" or "Dr. Joseph Smith, D/B/A Therapy Associates." Most banks require such certificates before an account is opened in a company name.

As a sole proprietor, a therapist may operate his practice as though it were a separate entity, although from a tax and financial viewpoint he is liable for all its obligations. His income is considered a *draw,* not salary. In fact, no member of the therapist's immediate family can receive a salary from a sole proprietorship.

On or before April 15th of each year, the practitioner must complete Schedule C of his IRS Form 1040. This is a profit-or-loss statement of the business.*

Partnerships

A partnership is an extension of a sole proprietorship. It is unincorporated, with partners sharing financial responsibility and profits according to a prearranged agreement. Every year an IRS Form 1065 (U.S. Partnership Return of In-

---

*If the business is set up on a fiscal instead of a calendar year, filing must take place on the fifteenth day of the fourth month after the close of the fiscal year. Most practitioners do not become involved in such arrangements unless specifically advised by an accountant or tax attorney.

come) must be filed on or before April 15th.* This is an informational return, since partnerships are not directly subject to income tax. Rather, each partner must report his share of the partnership income or loss when filing his personal return (Form 1040).

Corporations

The purposes of incorporating are to reduce financial liability and to take advantage of corporate tax deductions. However, incorporating does not always guarantee savings and in the final analysis, the advice of a tax attorney or accountant is necessary.

All corporations regardless of size, are similar in their essential characteristics. Corporations are owned by stockholders who elect a board of directors who control the corporation.† The IRS treats corporations as a separate tax entity. Because corporations are treated as individuals, their profits are subject to taxation. The therapist/owner of a corporation is paid wages by the corporation. These wages are, of course, also subject to state and federal taxation. The double tax situation can sometimes work to the therapist's disadvantage.

However, corporations may deduct certain expenses from taxable income that individuals may not deduct. Also, a corporation may employ its owner and his family. For example, the therapist's spouse can be employed by the corporation as bookkeeper. With a spouse as employee, the family may become eligible for personal tax deductions, such as childcare, to which it would not otherwise be entitled. Corporations may also deduct medical insurance and other fringe benefits paid for employees.

There are several types of corporate structures. In some states, professional corporations are designed specifically for professional practices. They are relatively easy to establish but may be restricted regarding size and principals. Another

*See footnote on preceeding page.
†The practitioner may be the sole stock owner, president and chairman of the board of his corporation.

type of corporation, the Small Business Corporation or Sub Chapter S, offers many of the advantages of the personally-owned and corporately-owned business.

Because the corporation is a legal entity, its owner has reduced financial liability. If the corporation disbands leaving debts, creditors have no recourse against the owners. However, such liability limitations are not boundless. The therapist is still liable for malpractice and if he personally co-signs a note or loan for the corporation, he will be held accountable.

TAXES

The kinds of taxes a practitioner pays depends on whether or not he has salaried employees and whether or not he is incorporated. If he is not incorporated and has no employees, his tax obligation is simpler.

Self-Employment Tax

This is Social Security tax as it applies to self-employed individuals of unincorporated businesses. The maximum figure one must pay has increased over the years. In 1977 the rate of tax was 8.1% of the net profits, with $16,500 the maximum taxable income. If a practitioner is salaried at another job where social security tax is deducted, his salary may be deducted from his private practice profits before self-employment tax is computed. For example, if a therapist works at North County Mental Health Clinic in addition to owning a private practice, his self-employment tax would be computed as follows:

Private Practice Income (maximum eligibility in 1977)	$16,500
Less Mental Health Clinic	15,900
Maximum applicable to self-employment tax	$ 600

In the above case, he would only have to pay a self-employment tax based on a percentage of the $600 figure, not on the full $16,500 earned in private practice. If a practitioner is incorporated, he is not subject to self-employment tax.

Social Security Tax

The full name for social security tax is the Federal Insurance Contributions Act and is usually referred to as FICA taxes. An employer must deduct a percentage of his employees wages as FICA tax. In addition, he must contribute to the government an equal amount of money. (This necessitates an employer identification number obtainable by filling out Form SS-4 at an IRS office). In 1977, the FICA tax was 5.85%, meaning that both the employer and employee made a combined contribution of 11.70 of wages up to a set limit. A therapist who is incorporated therefore, has to provide the entire contribution toward his own social security. Depending on the amount withheld, FICA is deposited on specific dates at any Federal Reserve Bank. The deposits are made with Form 501, available from any IRS office. It is absolutely critical to save the receipt, since it is the only bona fide proof of deposit. IRS will not accept a canceled check as proof of payment.

Income Tax Withholding

All wages are subject to income tax. However, unlike FICA, the percentage of income tax varies according to the amount of wages and number of dependents. Circular E, a free book of tables available at IRS offices can assist in computation. The amounts withheld are deposited along with the FICA.

Estimated Federal Income Tax

The sole proprietor of an unincorporated business is not paid wages but takes money or draws out of the business.

Draw is not subject to withholding taxes but the IRS insists that in such cases, income tax is paid in advance every 3 months. Taxes are estimated from past and anticipated earnings and must be filed on form 1040-ES by April 15, June 15, September 15, and January 15 of each year. The manner of estimating these taxes is complex, and is best left to a competent accountant. A fine is imposed for late filing.

Other Taxes, Contributions, and Penalties

Employers and the self-employed may also be subject to federal and state corporate profits tax and unemployment insurance contributions. The IRS and state taxation departments expect employers and the self-employed to be prompt in their deposits. Late payments invariably result in fines. Tax due dates should be marked on the calendar. Publication 334, *Tax Guide for Small Business*, provides detailed information about the topics discussed above, as well as clearly written interpretations of tax law. A good accountant is also extremely helpful in clarifying tax questions.

Tax Audits

On page 184 of Publication 334, the IRS says:

The vast majority of taxpayers are honest and have nothing to fear from an examination of their tax returns. An examination of such a taxpayer's return does not suggest a suspicion of dishonesty or criminal liability. It may not even result in more tax. Many cases are closed without change in reported tax liability and, in many others, the taxpayer receives a refund.

Notification of an audit comes in a polite computer-printed letter that describes audit procedure and what records are necessary to bring. The auditor will probably be as courteous and pleasant as a state patrolman giving a speeding ticket. Returns are selected for audit if blatant errors are found, or if selected by the computerized Discriminant Function System (DIF), or if randomly selected by the Taxpayer Compliance Measurement Program (TCMP). DIF assigns weights to various entries to aid in determining returns that have a high probability of errors. TCMP is a program designed to "measure and evaluate taxpayer compliance."

Audit questions may involve validity of receipts or valid records of items declared; eligibility to receive deductions declared; and earnings greater than the amount declared.

Because the IRS is often persistent and unyielding, many small businessmen unwisely give up without a fight even if their declarations are justified. Once the IRS succeeds in an audit, the chances are good that they will reaudit in the future. If an error is caught by the IRS, it is best to take the consequences and pay back taxes and fines. If one has been caught with a gross impropriety (such as not filing a return in 2 years), he had better hire a good lawyer.

Although only about two or three percent of returns are audited, an audit is always a possibility. If adequate records are kept, as outlined in Chapters 5 and 6, there should be no difficulty in proving claims for legitimate deductible items.

7 CLINICAL RECORDS*

*[This chapter was written by D. Robert Fowler, M.D.—R.M.P.]

This chapter gives practical advice on documenting treatment. Clinical programs frequently give little attention to training the intern or resident in the preparation of usable clinical records. Proper documentation is particularly critical to the private mental health practitioner who is solely responsible for his own performance.

PURPOSES AND FUNCTIONS

The purposes of clinical records are to:
1) serve as a basis for the planning and for the continuity of patient care;
2) provide a means of communication between the mental health professionals contributing to the patient's response to treatment;

3) document treatments and observations of the patient's response to treatment;
4) serve as a basis for review, study and evaluation of patient care;
5) assist in protecting the legal rights of therapist and patients;
6) serve as a basis for evaluating the clinical aspects of the practice.

The clinician who fails to keep adequate clinical records may be doing a disservice to his patients and missing an opportunity to learn more about them and about his practice. Maintaining adequate clinical records is worth the time it entails.

Maintaining records should help the clinician formulate his own thoughts about what is bothering the patient. Such documentation should record the clinician's plan for treatment and provide information by which the clinician can measure the patient's progress or lack of it in response to that treatment. The clinician, as well as the patient, is capable of distorting information that has not been recorded. A written account helps keep the clinician honest in terms of measuring the results of his evaluation and treatment.

Clinical documentation is also important because of the increased public accountability of mental health professionals. Records of treatment decisions and methods document the clinician's competence in cases reviewed by his peers, justify treatment for patients eligible for health insurance reimbursement, and can serve as evidence in trial cases or compensation hearings.

PROCESS NOTES

The most common form of record keeping is process notes, or case notes. Process notes are used by psychodynamically-oriented psychotherapists to retain information for their own use. One purpose of process notes, which are recorded during or immediately after an interview, is to allow the clinician to evaluate the process of the psychotherapeutic interchange, noting important themes possibly overlooked in the moment-to-moment psychotherapeutic interaction. Process notes contain very intimate and confidential information about the patient, as well as verbal interventions, questions and clarifying remarks made by the therapist. Process notes are valuable to the clinician only for a brief period of time. They have major shortcomings as documentation for permanent records.

The sheer volume of information contained in process notes makes them unlikely to be of value over a long period of time. Their intimate and confidential nature makes them unsuitable for communication to others. Process notes communicate little about the clinician's understanding of the case, his treatment plan, or the patient's response to treatment. Although they can be valuable for reviewing the previous two or three psychotherapy sessions, they do not record enough essential information to justify their use as clinical records. However, the essential information contained in process notes can be summarized, in regular progress notes and the process notes themselves then destroyed.

Finding Time

Special times must be allocated for adequate record keeping. Process notes should be recorded as soon after a session as possible. As in reporting dreams, a lapse of time is likely to result in embellishments of or deviations from the original content. So with case notes, the longer the delay in recording, the more likely they are to reflect something of the therapist's rather than the patient's personality. Secondly, postponing the recording of case notes increases the risk of the notes not being recorded at all. In time the therapist may not remember whether or not a particular note was dictated, and checking back to the charts may be inconvenient.

Most therapists prefer to record process notes chronologically using a page until it is filled. Recording one session on a page, tends to make a chart bulky. Also the order of such notes may get altered, and the absence of one page may not be readily missed.

If the notes are to be dictated, a pad of paper can be kept next to the dictating machine with the names of the patients entered when dictation begins. Thus, when the notes are transcribed all the necessary files can be retrieved in a single trip.

CONVENTIONAL VS. PROBLEM-ORIENTED RECORD SYSTEM

Depending upon their orientation, clinicians consider different data critical in the treatment of patients. No attempt is made here to suggest that one methodology or orientation is better than another. However, most practitioners will agree that treatment must be related to documentable observations or hypotheses. Certainly, most insurance companies demand such documentation for reimbursing patients or clinicians.

Both the conventional and the problem-oriented record system are discussed below. Either system, if properly documented, will be valuable to the therapist. Brevity and consiseness are important in both systems.

Identifying Information

Regardless of the type of records kept, certain identifying information is necessary. The identifying information, which can be kept separately from the principal record on a 3″ x 5″ file card, should include the patient's name and complete address, home and work telephone numbers, birthdate and age, sex, name and phone of nearest relative, the name of the person referring the patient, and information related to insurance coverage. Easy access to this information is critical in an emergency or if an appointment needs to be changed or cancelled. In addition, the patient's age, sex, marital status and referral source should also appear on the principal clinical record.

Conventional Record

Initial Evaluation. The first essential in the clinical record is the Initial Evaluation and Treatment Plan. The information in this part of the record may be derived from the first interview or, depending on the patient and the purposes of the evaluation, from several interviews. The major components in the initial evaluation and treatment plan are:

1. Identifying information (as indicated above);
2. Identification and development of the present problem(s) and pertinent related data;
3. The clinician's assessment of the patient's current problem(s) and level of functioning;
4. An initial plan that includes goals and means of treatment.

The information contained in the case history will depend strongly on the practitioner's conceptual framework. For example, the clinician who uses a strictly diagnostic approach finds certain information essential as part of the data base (case history), while the clinician who uses a strictly psychodynamic approach finds other information essential. The following suggested minimal components of the Initial Evaluation and Treatment Plan fit both conceptual models.

Presenting Problem and Related Data. The problem that brings the patient to therapy should be stated in his own words, if possible. The record should also note the referral source or how the patient came to therapy. In developing information related to the presenting problem the therapist should record important related data, including the time of onset of the problem, and its relationship to other life events, and whether the problem has occurred previously. In case, of previous occurrence, the relationship to life events should also be recorded, as well as whether treatment was provided and the nature of and response to treatment. The record should state whether the problem is continuous or episodic.

Depending upon the type of presenting problem, the presence or absence of related problems should be explored. Evidence of the presence or absence of alcohol or drugs should be noted, as well as evidence of any current medical problem and the physician treating it.

The effect of the problem(s) on significant areas in the patient's life should be documented. These areas include work or school, family relationships, social relationships, and leisure time activities. It should be noted whether the problem has resulted in difficulty for the patient in the community (e.g., has he been arrested?). This information will indicate how disabled the patient is by the presenting problem(s) and serve as a data set by which the clinician can judge changes in the patient's condition in response to treatment. In addition, documentation of the patient's current level of mental and emotional functioning (a mental status examination) is important. The patient's own understanding of the problem (insight) should be stated, using quotes if possible.

And finally, since there is a strong interrelationship between physical and emotional health, indication should be given regarding the patient's current physical health.

If there is doubt about the patient's physical health, the therapist should document his recommendations to the patient regarding further exploration of physical symptomatology.

Clinical Assessment. The identifying information and the case history should be as free from hypotheses as possible. The assessment will depend strongly on the clinician's theoretical orientation, his level of training and experience, and his willingness to commit himself on paper. Depending on theoretical orientation, the assessment section may include a diagnosis, a psychodynamic formulation, an interactional or transactional analysis, or a combination of these. The clinical assessment is a hypothesis connecting the problems of the patient with the clinician's treatment plan. It is an essential portion of the initial evaluation and treatment plan. By documenting his hypothesis and his plans for treatment, the clinician will improve his understanding of his patients and, ultimately, of his practice.

The assessment should attempt to explain why the patient has these problems at this particular time in his life. If the therapist is unable to explain certain problems, this fact should be stated. The clinician may say, for example, that without further information, he cannot explain particular symptoms or problems.

The Plan. This section of the initial evaluation and treatment plan should include plans for further evaluation and/or treatment. If further evaluation is necessary, the specific areas to be explored should be stated. Plans for treatment should include goals as well as the type and frequency of treatments planned.

The initial evaluation and treatment plan is not just an exercise in documenting information. The process of documenting hypotheses, goals and reasons for treatment is an exercise that clarifies the clinician's own thinking and leads to better evaluation and treatment. For this reason, the initial evaluation and treatment plan is probably the most essential part of the clinical record.

Progress Notes. Progress notes summarize patient's present status, the treatment being provided, and the patient's response to these treatments. Regular progress notes afford the clinician an opportunity to review his own thinking about the patient. These notes should record changes in plans, changes in the patient's status, and changes in frequency and type of treatment.

The frequency of recording progress notes depends on how often the patient is seen, and also on his condition. For example, a crisis such as increased suicidal risk should be documented in a progress note. In such instances the clinician should record the events and his assessment of their significance, alternatives for intervention, and his rationale for selecting an alternative. (For an example of format, see Appendix.)

Discharge or Termination Notes. When treatment is terminated, the clinician should document the course of treatment in a termination note. This note should briefly review the patient's status at the time of initial evaluation; the clinician's assessment of the patient at that time and his plans for treatment; the treatment provided; the patient's response to treatment; and the clinician's final assessment and recommendations for follow-up. Properly and concisely written, this note can be used to transmit information to appropriate mental health professionals or to the referral source. (For an example of format, see Appendix.)

The Problem-Oriented Record System

An alternative system for keeping clinical records, which involves identifying the separate problems or symptoms presented by the patient, carefully describing each problem and maintaining a separate assessment and plan for each identified problem, is called the problem-oriented record system (Weed, 1970; Fowler and Longabaugh, 1975; Grant and Maletski, 1972; Ryback, 1974). Proponents of this system maintain that it increases the comprehensiveness of patient evaluation and treatment and contributes to improved patient care by documenting the patient's progress and responses to specific treatments in an orderly and systematic fashion. Many practitioners assert that this system facilitates an interdisciplinary approach to patient care and makes quality review and program planning more accessible. The following is a synopsis of the essential features of the system. (An example of the use of this system is seen in the Appendix.)

The essential components of the problem-oriented record system are:
1. The data base;
2. The problem list;
3. The initial plan;
4. The progress notes.

Data Base. The data base consists of the patient's case history and includes information from the patient and the clinician's observations. The case history is similar to that kept in a traditional record, with the information presented as free from hypotheses and assessments as possible.

Problem List. From the data base, the clinician identified problems affecting the patient. These problems are assembled into a numbered list which serves as an index and table of contents for the rest of the clinical record.

Initial Plan. The initial plan consists of a description, assessment and plan for each problem on the numbered problem list. As in the initial evaluation and treatment plan of the conventional record, the assessment includes the clinician's hypotheses about the origin of the patient's problems in terms of a diagnosis, a dynamic formulation and/or transactional analysis, depending on the clinician's theoretical orientation. In the case of the problem-oriented record system, however, an assessment is made of each problem, although the assessments of several problems may be interrelated. (See Appendix.)

Although the information in the plan of the problem-oriented record system is similar to that in the traditional record, this system includes a plan for each problem. All treatments are coded to the problem for which they are provided.

Progress Notes. Progress notes are written regularly for each problem. In outpatient practice, progress notes summarize the current status of each problem following the format of description, assessment and plan. (See Appendix.) Additional progress notes recording a crisis or important change (for example, a suicide risk), may concern only a single problem.

Termination Note. The termination note, written in the problem-oriented format, includes for each numbered problem a summary of its description; its course during treatment; the types of treatment provided; the patient's response to treatment; future plans, if any. (See Appendix.)

The problem-oriented record system has advantages

over the traditional record system in terms of comprehensiveness of documentation. It is more efficient in pointing up major omissions of assessment and treatment planning. However, many clinicians feel that the problem-oriented record system requires too much time to justify its use on a regular basis.

RECORDS AND ACCOUNTABILITY

In the past the public has been satisfied with efforts by the mental health profession to assure the competence and ethics of its members. Recent changes on the national scene indicate that at least some of the public is not satisfied with such intraprofessional monitoring. For example, the Social Security Amendments of 1972 (Public Law 92-603) establishes a system of Professional Standards Review Organizations whose function is to monitor the cost and quality of health care. This and other recently enacted laws are seen as precursors to a comprehensive national health insurance program which will to some extent finance mental health services. Explicit in these laws are provisions for public accountability.

Current procedures for reviewing mental health services rely primarily on information provided in clinical records. Current practice includes review by non-professional "claims reviewers" and by committees composed of professional peers. Although emphasis has been on reviewing in-hospital services, provisions have already been made for similar reviews of outpatient mental health services. Such provisions have given impetus to the recent emphasis on improving the quality of clinical records. Most independent mental health practitioners are now, or will soon be, subjected to the following review procedures:

1. Claim review;
2. Peer review;

3. Utilization review.

These review procedures monitor quality and cost of care provided by mental health practitioners. They place considerable importance on adequate clinical records as a reflection of the quality of treatment.

Claims Review

"Claims review" is a term used by health insurance companies to describe the review of clinical records to determine whether the services provided are eligible for reimbursement by the insurance company; whether the services provided were necessary; whether the services provided and the cost of such services were appropriate and within reasonable limits.

Some health insurance companies do not provide coverage for mental health services. Others cover only those mental health services provided by a physician. Still others cover services provided by mental health professionals under the supervision of a physician, and a few cover services provided by other qualified mental health professionals. If the insurance contract covers his services, the clinician should be able to document that the patient's problems were evaluated, appropriate treatment was planned and provided, and the type and frequency of treatment was necessary and acceptable according to local practice and standards. These issues can be documented in a letter to the insurance company without specifying potentially embarrassing or damaging information. Claims containing only necessary information stand a better chance of being approved. Mental health jargon, intimate details and long histories only distract from the necessary decision making. Adequate clinical records make composing such a letter relatively simple.

If a claim that the therapist believes justified is denied, he can request a peer-review decision from his professional organization, provided that his organization has such a procedure.

Peer Review

Many professional organizations provide peer review services on a voluntary basis. Although some peer review committees of professional societies serve on ethical questions, most committees consider cases dealing with appropriateness of treatment. Such cases can be referred to peer review committees by patients, clinicians, health insurance companies, or hospitals, to determine whether services provided were necessary; appropriate in terms of treatment; of adequate quality; appropriate in terms of frequency and cost.

A peer review committee may request a copy of clinical records or a letter from the clinician explaining his evaluation and treatment. Such committees, composed of mental health professionals, are bound by the same ethics of confidentiality as the clinician himself. It is advisable, however, to have the patient's written permission before providing a copy of his record to a peer review committee.

If the clinician has documented his evaluation and treatment according to the guidelines outlined in this chapter, the peer review committee should have no difficulty in making a determination.

Utilization Review

Utilization review is an interdisciplinary review procedure used to monitor services and determine whether they were necessary, appropriate, and the least expensive form of treatment necessary for the patient's condition. This form of monitoring currently takes place in a hospital setting, where a utilization review committee regularly reviews clinical records to determine whether the hospital is being efficiently and appropriately utilized. Plans are currently being made to extend utilization review procedures into outpatient practice. Again, clinical records or a summary of clinical records will probably be the way in which utilization review committees monitor the quality and cost of outpatient treatment.

RECORDS AND CONFIDENTIALITY

A foundation of the mental health profession is the principle of confidentiality. Breaches of confidentiality may range from the simple revelation that a person is receiving treatment to the revelation of potentially embarrassing and damaging information. Without the assurance of confidentiality and privacy, crucial information may be withheld by the patient. The issue of confidentiality is not confined to clinical records, but written information is more accessible to breaches of confidentiality.

Every precaution must be taken to preserve confidentiality and to guard against attempts by others to breach these precautions. The therapist must very carefully assess the legitimacy of requests for information about patients, and should release no information without the patient's written consent. Unless clinically contraindicated, the patient should be informed concerning the content of material for which he is asked to sign a release. Therapists should be aware of the practice of some health insurance companies of obtaining blanket permission for release of information, even prior to services being rendered. Such signed releases should be considered invalid for releasing confidential information.

Schools, potential employers and others may request information pertaining to a patient's ability to function in a particular situation. Such requests place the clinician in an uncomfortable position. If he does not comply, the patient may be denied the opportunity he seeks. If he does comply, even with the patient's permission, potentially embarrassing information may be revealed. In such circumstances, the therapist can state that the patient was being seen for reasons other than an evaluation of job or school ability and that another clinician should see the patient in order to make that a determination.

Telephone inquiries are somewhat more difficult to handle. The therapist might reply that he never gives out information over the telephone and can not even say if the person mentioned is or is not his patient.

Case records should be kept in a locked filing cabinet, preferably in the therapist's office. Although such precautions do not insure complete protection, they at least make it more difficult for confidentiality to be violated.

GROUP PRIVATE PRACTICE*

*[*Written with Frank D. E. Jones, M.D.—R.M.P.*]

THE CONCEPT

Group private practice is an enterprise in which more than one practitioner provides services at a single location. The enterprise may be a partnership, a sole proprietorship employing others, or a corporation consisting of two or more principals. As individual private practice has its lure, so does group private practice. Occasionally novice therapists band together to begin a practice; sometimes more experienced therapists attempt to expand a practice by hiring another practitioner.

The beginner dreams of safety in numbers; the experienced therapist hopes for additional income. A well-run group practice seems attractive, but unless handled carefully, such attempts can be disastrous. This caution is not meant to discourage clinicians from group practice but to simply note that it is more difficult to formulate and maintain a successful group practice than an individual one. With careful planning and avoidance of common pitfalls, a group practice can be stimulating and financially rewarding.

The Pitfalls

Certain problems arise when beginning practitioners open group practices. Frequently there are not enough referrals to go around, thus creating anxiety about financial stability. If employee therapists are expected to promote referrals, they may feel they have a share in the ownership of the practice. Yet from a legal viewpoint, the feeling of ownership is unjustified and may result in disappointment and confusion. Problems regarding finance and ownership are so critical that if not handled effectively, endless misunderstandings may absorb the energies of all involved. Insufficient referrals can also result in jealousy and competition. Also, if the employer-therapist is ambivalent regarding each person's role (including his own) in the practice, confusion and bad feelings can result.

Sole Ownership vs. Shared Ownership

There are two types of mental health group private practices: one owned by an individual, the other owned by two or more individuals. Individual ownership is less potentially difficult than shared ownership which usually occurs among beginning practitioners and can be fraught with misunderstandings. However, it is not impossible to have a successful shared practice.

SOLE OWNERSHIP

When To Start

Some introspection is worthwhile before any such major change as the move from an individual to a group practice. Owning a group practice increases one's work rather than reduces it. Although there is the opportunity to augment one's salary considerably, there are also more problems, pressures, and responsibilities. Managerial skills and financial expertise are needed, and constant effort must be made to insure a steady influx of referrals.

A group practice should be embarked upon only when one is financially and professionally stable. Forming a group practice is a poor way to create such stability. Most successful group practice owners add personnel only after the demand is indicated. A consistent 20% to 25% work overload would indicate the need for an additional staff member. If a therapist feels that 30 hours a week is an ideal caseload, an increase to about 36 hours a week would justify a staff addition. Usually staff is hired on a parttime basis for blocks of five or ten hours. Since most employees will have other affiliations with a hospital, clinic, or university, they might be available only at evening or weekend hours. Since the therapist-employer must be present when they are working (for reasons explained later), their available hours will be a critical factor in hiring.

Wages and Fees

Many group practices pay wages according to the number of contact hours the therapists has with patients. Wages should not be contingent on collections from patients. The wage should be set at an hourly rate that is attractive to the employee and fiscally sound for the employer-therapist. The wage should be commensurate with the therapist's training and skill.

Patient's fees need not vary according to the therapist they see. Since the employer-therapist is responsible for the delivery of services and the care of all patients, and all employees work under his supervision and direction, fees to patients should be uniform. One psychiatrist, who charges at the 90th percentile for half hour sessions with either himself or staff, pays his therapists from one third to two thirds of the fee, depending on training and experience. His employees have no overhead expenses and earn a guaranteed wage, dependent only on contact hours (amply supplied by the psychiatrist) and not on collections. Payment of two thirds of the fee is unusually generous and undoubtedly contributes to the stability of this psychiatrist's staff.

Rather than pay an employee-therapist a wage subject to standard tax deductions, many employers pay a consultant's fee on the basis of the number of hours worked. There are a number of reasons for paying this way. Since the amount of pay might vary from week to week, deductions would also vary and require unwieldy bookkeeping. Standard wages also requires more extensive bookkeeping procedures and necessitates employer contribution to social security. This practice is widespread and frequently recommended by tax attorneys.

In order to qualify as consultants, therapists must be licensed, certified or otherwise qualified for independent practice. They provide services under the employer-therapist's but are responsible for paying their own taxes. An accountant or tax attorney can advise further on this issue and may recommend a special consultant's contract. Chapter 9 further discusses the difference between a consultant and employee, and may be helpful in determining which method of payment is most applicable to a particular practice.

Even though a consultant arrangement may be simpler and slightly less expensive for the employer, it may cause ambiguity for the therapists concerning their roles as employees. Paying standard wages better satisfies the spirit of the law and better defines employee relations.

Who Is In Charge

It must be clear to staff and patients that the practice belongs to the employer-therapist. He has final responsibility for all clinical and business matters. While the staff should be highly competent and able to make independent clinical judgements or know when to seek consultation, the employer-therapist must be responsible for all decisions concerning the management of the practice, its policies, the manner of communicating with referral sources, allocation of patients, and setting of wages. He can and often should seek consultation with staff, but the final decisions are his.

Hiring Staff

Most group practices are composed of part-time employees. However, full-time employment occasionally evolves over a period of time. There is an advantage in knowing employees well before hiring them, although this is not always possible. Selecting a therapist is more complicated and more critical than selecting nonprofessional staff. If it is necessary to recruit staff, the methods explained in Chapter 9 may be helpful. In order to provide clinical, medical, or administrative supervision, the employer-therapist must be present when staff is working. Therefore, hours of availability are a critical consideration in hiring, second only to compatibility and qualifications.

Some employers prefer a written contract with employees while others do not. There is certainly no harm in having a written contract. If nothing else, it provides the opportunity to spell out mutual expectations and responsibilities. When personnel are previously unknown, a written contract is certainly advisable. Hiring procedures are discussed in more detail in Chapter 9.

Patient Management

Intake Interview. The employer-therapist should do all intake interviews. Since physicians and others make referrals to him, they expect him to see the patient. If the referred patient is first seen by someone else, both the patient and the referral source may feel slighted. Referrals made within the practice, as described later, should not offend referrer or patient. Also, doing intakes allows the employer-therapist to do the initial diagnosis or diagnostic hypothesis and to make the appropriate referral within the practice. This is the first step in establishing the employer's overall clinical responsibility in the practice. The intake interview establishes a tie between the employer and each patient, permitting him to orient each patient and to intervene later in the therapy if appropriate. Such intervention may be necessary if a patient stops paying his bill.

Two procedures are important in intake interviews. First, the assessment must be written up promptly so that it can be used for intra-office referral. Either the conventional or data based format discussed in Chapter 7 can be used. Second, the employer must set aside a time not ordinarily used for therapy to do intakes. If intakes are done during regular therapy hours, the therapist is likely to find himself underemployed during those times when intakes drop off.

Intra-Office Referrals. As the sole intake worker, the employer-therapist has the responsibility for helping the patient make a comfortable transition from himself to one of the other therapists. It is best to indicate to each patient at the onset that he himself will be seeing the patient a few times to assess which therapist will be best for him. The explanations should be presented in a positive way, pointing out, for example, that some individuals work best with a male or female therapist, or that a particular therapist may be more in tune with certain problems. It is helpful to provide the patient with a brief assessment of his problem and the reason for assigning him to a particular therapist. However, the patient should always feel that he has a choice and that the decision is not irreversible. If, for example, the patient insists on seeing the employer-therapist, he may be put on his waiting list and/or assigned to another therapist until he is available. Also, if clinically indicated, patients may be reassigned to other therapists as therapy progresses. Obviously, this should not be done when transference is a major aspect of the therapeutic processes. To some degree, transference and countertransference are de-emphasized in group practice. Of course, if a patient wishes to change therapists (or vice versa) in the middle of therapy, transference issues should be examined. However, an intra-office referral may prevent termination when a patient's therapy becomes stagnated.

Office Procedures

Telephone Service. A group practice needs two or more telephone lines. One telephone line per therapist plus an additional line free for incoming calls should be adequate. While lines should be added conservatively, a practitioner may be held liable for malpractice if it is found that he has not made himself sufficiently available to seriously ill patients.

It is essential that part-time therapists can be easily reached. If a practice involves more than two therapists, it is unwieldy for the answering service to have them all check in frequently. It is best to type out a simple schedule for the service so they know where each therapist can be reached in an emergency. Only the employer or the receptionist then, will check in with the service.

Scheduling Therapists. To facilitate supervision and referrals, the employer should begin his sessions five minutes later than the other therapists. This permits him to use the last five minutes of his session to introduce a patient to his new therapist after intake. Also, this framework permits a psychiatrist-employer to provide medication consultation for the other therapists.

Each therapist must be responsible for maintaining two appointment books, one kept by him and the other by the receptionist. For reasons explained later, a receptionist is almost always needed for a group practice. If there is no receptionist, the employer should keep the second, or master, appointment book. Whenever a therapist adds or drops an appointment, the change should be entered in both books, thus enabling the employer to schedule patients after intake interviews. If these books are not kept current, the probability of double-scheduling and other confusion increases.

Clinical Records. Good clinical records are particularly important in a group practice. Either traditional or data-based records, as discussed in Chapter 7, can be used. Records are one method by which staff can communicate to the employer about patient progress and therapy planning. Individual supervision, as outlined later, is another method. Well-kept clinical records greatly increase the value of supervision. The employer is, legally and for insurance purposes, liable for all the patients. The records are one way of establishing his involvement with them, particularly if he initials the records when he examines them.

In order to insure that records are kept current, every effort should be made to facilitate record keeping for the staff. For a small group practice, individual recorders with a transcriber for the typist might be made available. For groups of four or more therapists, a communication system consisting of two or more recorders located at the typist's desk and microphones located in each therapist's offices is recommended. When a therapist wishes to dictate, the microphone automatically transfers to an available machine. The expense of such equipment must be weighed against savings in secretarial costs.

A policy should be established regarding clinical records. Therapists can be asked to keep process notes after each session and to condense these notes into progress notes at least every two months. A prompt termination note will enable the employer to communicate with the referral sources when necessary and appropriate. The termination note is particularly critical if a patient requests that information to be forwarded after termination.

Collection of Fees and Billing. All checks should be made payable to the employer-therapist. If there is a receptionist, fees are usually collected by him. Patient traffic should be routed so that all patients pass the receptionist when they leave.

It is best to encourage patients to pay as they go, particularly in a group practice. There is always the possibility that employed therapists will be lax with patients who fall behind in payments. If patients are allowed to pay monthly, it will take longer for the employer to become aware of payment problems. The receptionist or a therapist should alert the employer to patients who fall behind, thus giving him the opportunity to intervene directly. He should not hesitate to tell the patient that fees must be collected to pay therapists salaries and other costs, and that for therapy to continue the fee must be paid or some satisfactory arrangement agreed upon. Sometimes a patient who has fallen behind can pay an additional $5 each session until he has caught up. Some therapists offer patients the option of going into group therapy during financial hard times. Lack of payment then is not as costly to the therapist.

Bills should always go out on the employer's letterhead. A code system can be used to designate each therapist. The use of his letterhead emphasizes the employer's role as chief clinician in the practice.

Supervision. In a group practice where therapists are employees, supervision is necessary both legally and clinically. Most employers agree that employees should receive at least one hour of face-to-face supervision for every six hours of therapy delivered. Some feel the ratio should be one hour for every three hours of therapy. Generally, one hour of supervision is recommended for each group session. The need for supervision will vary according to the training of the employees and the type of caseloads they carry. However, unless specific time is set aside for supervision on a regular basis, it is likely to be haphazard and ineffective.

Continuing Education. Employees should be encouraged to learn new skills and improve old ones. Periodic workshops or seminars vitalize individual therapists and the practice as a whole. While it is not equitable to demand that employees attend continuing education programs, they can be given incentives in the form of verbal praise or a monetary bonus. Periodically, therapists can be allowed to share or teach their skills at staff meetings. However, unless they are paid for their attendance, such meetings, if held too frequently, will be resented.

ALTERNATE GROUP PRACTICES

Corporations and Partnerships

An alternate form of group practice is a partnership in which ownership is shared by two or more therapists. There are several inherent pitfalls in partnerships. Decisions must be shared and frequently compromised. Problems arise when one partner seems to work harder, or draws more clientele, or spends more company resources than the other. However, some partnerships thrive and such an operation must be considered a viable option. The advantage of a partnership is that such expenses as rent, utilities, telephone and answering service can be shared.

Potential partners must first find a location that can support two or more mental health practitioners. The following course can then be taken.

A corporation can be formed to take care of the business aspects of the practice. (For explanation of how a corporation works, see Chapter 9). The corporation then rents the office, telephone, and answering service to the therapists. Although the corporation controls the business, each therapist maintains control over and responsibility for his own practice.

A lawyer should set up the corporation, but the following is a brief description of how it might work. Dr. Whitney and Dr. Smith, through their corporation, secure a fully-equipped office with two therapy rooms, a reception and waiting room. Both therapists go about the business of promoting their practices as indicated in Chapter 4. Each month the corporation bills them for their relative share of expenses. (See facing page).

Incorporation is not essential if a similar arrangement can be worked out in a partnership. The primary advantage of incorporation is that individual liability is limited should the endeavor fail. In drafting an agreement, some provision should be made for dissolving the corporation if necessary and permitting either of the principals to purchase equip-

Office Expenses		Dr. Whitney's Share	Dr. Smith's Share
Rent	$200	$100	$100
Telephone	20	10	10
Toll Calls	30	26.30	3.70
Answering Service	30	15	15
Typist	260	180	80
Equipment Rental	90	45	45
Furniture Rental	95	47.50	47.50
Supplies	10	5	5
Administration of Corporation	35	17.50	17.50
Total	$770	$446.30	$323.70

ment if desired. A common arrangement provides that the remaining therapist take over payments for the equipment plus pay the therapist who is leaving half his original contribution.

Individual Identity in Partnerships

In this arrangement, each therapist preserves his own identity. The telephone should be answered, "Dr. Smith's and Dr. Whitney's office." Also, each therapist should have his own letterhead, billing system (although the labor may be shared) professional liability insurance (fire and theft, etc. can be shared) and clientele. A problem may arise if someone calls for an appointment and gives no preference for either therapist. Such contingencies should be carefully discussed and the solutions provided in writing.

Taking in a Partner

Sometimes a successful practitioner wants to take in a partner. Usually this is done either to secure capital or as a preliminary step in selling the practice. The sale of all or part of a mental health practice is a relatively new idea with little data available as a guideline. The following procedure is only done with highly successful, well-established practices.

The incoming partner agrees to purchase the practice from the established therapist for a percentage (sometimes as high as 100%) of one year's gross plus a percentage of the value of the equipment. The year's gross is first estimated by averaging three to five years of the established therapist's receipts, with the final amount based on an average of two to three years of the new therapist's receipts. The new therapist usually gives a 10% to 20% down payment with the remainder paid in equal installments over a four to ten year period. If the established therapist intends to retire, he may transfer his entire caseload to his new partner over a period of two to three years.

When therapists work in partnership, the costs of the operation are usually shared, with nearly all fees going to the therapist performing the work. Other arrangements are bound to produce misunderstandings.

Earnings

Successful group practice owners report that their net earnings range from 15% to 50% above their individual practice earnings. But it must be emphasized that extraordinary work is required to increase earnings to this degree. Time must be spent on such non-income producing activities as supervision, office management, and employee relations. In addition, considerable time must be spent in securing and maintaining referral sources. However, once established, a group practice can provide substantial financial stability for its owner, because in fact employees generate income at a rate that exceeds their salaries.

9   MAINTENANCE AND EXPANSION

A private practice needs to be constantly cultivated and nourished. As conditions change, so do strategies for keeping the practice healthy and productive. Less energy is required to maintain a practice than establish one, but even maintenance demands an absolute commitment. Expansion of a practice demands as much energy as the formulation of one.

MAINTAINING REFERRALS

Referral sources are the mainstay of a practice, and constant attention is necessary to maintain them. It is realistic to anticipate competition for referrals, but this needn't be a threat if strong lines of communication have been established between the therapist and his sources. Frequently, referrals fall off only because the source is not thinking of the therapist's services. The following strategies help to counteract this problem.

Feedback

Referral feedback is essential for both the advanced and beginning practitioner. When a source first refers an individual or family for therapy, it is natural for him to be concerned about his patients and wonder at least whether they have contacted the therapist. Even after a regular referral procedure is established, he will continue to have these concerns. The following feedback strategies are recommended.

Phone Call. The easiest, but not necessarily most effective method of feedback is to phone the referral source when the patient calls for an appointment. The purpose of the call is simply to inform the source that the appointment has been made. The effectiveness of such a call depends on the orientation of the referral source. Some doctors do not want more than minimal information and would consider long reports or telephone calls burdensome. However, a short call reinforces the referral source and often a second referral follows such a call.

Brief Letter. A brief letter to the referral source when the patient comes in for the appointment can be sent in lieu of phoning.

Dear Dr. Webb:

On your recommendation, your patient, Mr. Steven Apley came in today for an initial interview. It appears that a marital problem may exist, and I have asked him to return with Mrs. Apley next week. I will keep you abreast of the progress.

Thank you very much for referring this interesting young man to my office.

Sincerely,

Such a letter cannot ethically be sent without the patient's written permission. As a matter of course, the therapist might secure a *release of information* during the first interview in order to facilitate communication with the referral source. Naturally, the interests of patients come first. The therapist should not urge the signing of a release if a patient expresses reluctance, except if the referral is due to medically oriented complaints. Most patients will sign a release if one is routinely requested in the first interview, but later requests may be awkward or antitherapeutic.

Information in such a letter should be only enough to inform the referral source that the patient is receiving adequate attention and that he will be kept apprised of the patient's progress. Two key phrases are "Your patient" and "Thank you for referring." The first assures the referral source that his position is not being usurped. The second phrase recognizes the mutually beneficial relationship between the two practitioners.

Reports and Forms. The phone call or the letter should be used when the patient first calls or is seen. Subsequent methods of feedback serve several functions:

1. Coordination of treatment among practitioners.
2. Keeping lines of communication open.
3. Permitting the referral source to feel involved with treatment.
4. Educating the referral source regarding the practitioner's services.

Reports must be geared to the reader and be in the patient's best interest. No matter what safeguards the therapist employs, once confidential information leaves his office, he no longer has control over it. It is not unrealistic to expect that such information may eventually reach the patient.

Sometimes referral sources need or want detailed reports. A school referral often includes a request for specific information or recommendations. However, a short format is usually appropriate and sufficient. The data based report mentioned in Chapter 7 can be adapted for this purpose. Reports can be made even simpler by utilizing a preprinted form as shown in the appendix. This format permits the practitioner to write the note quickly in long hand, but still preserves a professional quality to the communication. It provides for a concise statement of diagnosis and treatment plan, the two items of primary interest to the referral source. Ethically however, the patient should be apprised of the extent and scope of such a report.

Case Conferences. Certain categories of referral sources, such as medical groups and schools, are particularly receptive to case conferences. The result is usually a better understanding of the case. The mechanics of setting up a conference may have to be established by the practitioner. Schools often lack a built in structure for organizing conferences but with some help from the administration, it is often possible to arrange for key staff members to meet. It is unrealistic to expect school personnel to give more time than an hour.

Much has been written about consultations and case conferences. The annotated bibliography lists several excellent books on these subjects. Two points regarding such meetings are worth mentioning here. First, the responsibility for presenting material should be shared. The therapist should ask others for observations and encourage elaboration. Second, some plan of action, even a simple one, should be established by the close of the meeting. If these two rules are followed, the referral sources will feel a sense of participation and purpose in the conference.

Announcements

Most practitioners send announcements to referral sources when they begin practice. However, announcements can be more effective if sent two to three years after the practice is established. Such an announcement would not follow the usual format, but should consist of a brief letter and material similar to that mentioned earlier. A communication of this type is especially appropriate if an initial announcement was never sent, or if services or personnel have been added. Repeated mailings, however, are inappropriate and may be rightfully construed as soliciting. The recipients should be carefully picked and exclude sources currently making referrals.

News Release

A practice almost always benefits from positive public exposure. Concise news releases can be sent to the local paper regarding such public-oriented activities as a committee or board appointment, conducting a school or community workshop, or even a social gathering that has significance in terms of mental health. Either the therapist or the sponsoring agency can provide copy for the newspaper. Items about committee appointments can be mailed to the newspaper's city desk. The editor might save the article for a few days and use it as a filler. Local community papers will sometimes print a short advance story about a workshop, especially if it is sponsored by a school or local community agency. A relaxation workshop offered by the local library or a workshop sponsored by the school district on improving parent-teacher relationships might be considered a good feature story.

Some therapists, particularly those beginning practice, are reluctant to send out press releases. However, if certain guidelines are observed, news releases should pose no compromise to ethics or modesty. First, the event publicized should be newsworthy and of public interest. It should be of public service or reflect unusual achievement. The release should not be an attempt to advertise services or routine business. The following are appropriate topics for a news release:

1. Delivery of workshops sponsored by public agencies
2. Receipt of award for outstanding achievement
3. Appointment to board or committee posts
4. Hosting a major social event, such as a reception for a new hospital director.

Format of News Release. The news release should be typed double-spaced on plain bond paper in the format shown below. The most important information should be presented at the beginning of the release. The report should be factual, with opinions attributed to their source. The therapist's name and phone number should appear at the bottom of the page for the purpose of verification. The following is a sample news release.

NEWS RELEASE

Special to Daily Times
(Today's date)

DR. ANDERSON APPOINTED TO COMMISSION

Governor Wm. T. Blackberry today announced the appointment of Charles J. Anderson, M.D. to the State Mental Health Commission. Dr. Anderson, a psychiatrist, is a resident of Larchmont and practices in Newfield.

The State Mental Health Commission was first formed in 1967 to oversee the State Mental Health Hospital network. Dr. Anderson's appointment completes a 23-person panel composed of mental health professionals throughout the state.

Dr. Anderson is on the faculty of the State University and is currently chairman of the university's forum on mental health. He is the author of several professional articles, as well as the recently-published text, *Psychiatry and the Community*.

Dr. Anderson said that he was honored by the Governor's appointment. "Continued upgrading of the State Mental Health Hospital network is my first priority," he said.

One needn't be intimidated by the size of the newspaper. Even the largest city newspapers need to fill space between the ads. A news release may find its way to page 78 of the *New York Times* as easily as to page 2 of the *Ashtabula Star Beacon*.

EXPANSION

Groups

Groups add a new dimension to a practice. Beginning therapists often have difficulty finding enough patients of the right mix for a therapeutic group, but the seasoned practitioner has a broader base of patients and referral sources from which to draw. Group therapy is very rewarding financially. If the therapist sees eight patients for 90 minutes at $15 per patient, he earns nearly $80 per hour.

Many practitioners feel that group therapy is particularly indicated for certain individuals or problems. Couples groups (marital therapy), young adult groups, adolescent groups and child activity groups are frequently offered by private clinicians.

From the standpoint of private practice, adequate space and collection of fees are the primary logistical problems in offering group therapy. Waiting rooms tend to become crowded and the noise level can rise. Fees should be collected by a receptionist, or billed biweekly to the patient. Having patients line up to pay the therapist before or after a session can be a demoralizing experience for all concerned.

Workshops

Workshops can be more than a public relations service. They can be an integral part of the therapist's work for which he receives regular income. Public schools are the most frequent workshop sponsors, particularly under federal or state-funded programs. The workshops may be intended for training or to meet other school program goals. Other workshop sponsors include municipal departments such as mental health, education, social welfare, public safety and justice. A good workshop often results in a request for a repeat performance. Industry is also often interested in sponsoring workshops.

Consultation

Providing services to industry or schools is another way of expanding a practice. In recent years, many industrial firms have become concerned about the mental health of their employees. Although many larger firms have staff trained to counsel employees in work-related problems, most do not. In order to be retained, a therapist must convince a firm that specific therapeutic services can increase productivity and profits. Alcohol counseling and rehabilitation programs have been sold to many industries because absenteeism drops when such programs are successfully instituted.

Schools often contract for mental health services. Smaller school districts in particular cannot readily hire full-time psychiatrists or psychologists in order to meet federal regulations. However, these districts can contract for specific amounts or types of services from private practitioners.

HIRING STAFF

In time, most practices evolve so that either office staff or professional staff need to be hired. Hiring personnel is a procedure that industry takes quite seriously. Not only does staff affect the efficiency of a practice, it also reflects on the therapist's professional image. In a field in which time and service are the commodities sold, the therapist's image in the community is quite critical.

Mental health employees usually fall into two categories: professional staff, usually designated as therapists; office staff, usually classified as secretarial, clerical, bookkeeping or a combination of the three.

Office Staff

Employees can constitute the single greatest overhead expense for the private practitioner. Every effort should be made to consolidate office work and avoid unnecessary hiring. When a practice is thriving, however, the full-time practitioner will have to hire at least a part-time secretary.

Recruitment. Although the duties of staff should be determined prior to hiring, most positions become more fully defined after staff is hired. This is particularly true for beginning therapists.

Recruitment procedure may greatly affect the quality of

staff. Despite training in personality assessment, mental health practitioners are not better equipped to select qualified staff than their counterparts in industry. In fact, most industrial enterprises have more logical hiring procedures than mental health practitioners. The following system is borrowed from industry and modified for application to private practice staff.

The five major sources of recruitment are word of mouth, selective advertising, state employment offices, professional employment agencies and professional schools. The first two methods place the greatest burden on the employer. The first method, though frequently used, is the most haphazard. Word of mouth is a nice way of keeping in touch with colleagues, but one should not expect to hire office staff using this method.

Before selecting a method, the therapist should know the qualifications he is seeking. Agencies and advertisements will not be able to discern such abstract qualities as "honesty, dedication, and intelligence." However, they can help find personnel who meet certain concrete requirements.

One to two years experience is very beneficial in office help, particularly for the beginning therapist who is in a poor position to train a secretary or a bookkeeper. The minimum typing speed required by state or government agencies is 40 words per minute. Typing should be relatively error-free. Experienced secretaries type more than 75 words per minute, with only one error in a 60-second test. Experience with dictating equipment is also helpful, as is familiarity with the specific type of equipment available in the therapist's office. However, most secretaries readily adapt to new equipment. Shorthand ability need not be required but it permits the therapist to dictate a letter directly to the secretary and also permits the secretary to take telephone notes more quickly.

Help wanted advertisements are placed in the classified section of the newspaper. Most newspapers permit ads to be called in. The ad should include qualifications, salary, and, of course, a return telephone number or address. Since the ad might elicit unqualified candidates, the therapist will have to do his own screening. Having candidates telephone facilitates the screening procedure considerably. The following questions might be used for screening:

1. Do you type at least 45 words per minute?
2. Are you available to work evening or weekend hours?
3. Would you consider a salary of $4.00 per hour?

Only candidates who answer all the questions affirmatively should be scheduled for an interview.

State employment services, private agencies and school placement services usually have a pool of potential candidates to be placed. They are particularly useful because they screen candidates according to the requirements of the job before sending them out. There are differences between these three placement agencies in screening. Private agencies charge a fee to either the employer or employee when their candidate is hired. Professional schools offer the best opportunity for recruiting secretarial staff since they specialize in office staff training. Graduates must meet minimum standards (which are quite adequate) and placement service is free.

A temporary office help agency supplies office staff on a day-to-day basis. If temporary help is used on a regular basis, much of the employer's time may be spend in training. In an emergency, however, it might be necessary to use temporary help. If the employer finds a particularly well-qualified temporary employee, the agency might release the employee to him for a fee, usually $200 to $300.

The Interview. Unless the therapist's background is in industrial psychology, it is unlikely that his interview technique will help in selecting a candidate. The purpose of the interview is to appraise the candidate's skills, validate the candidate's experience, and observe the candidate's appearance and demeanor. Volumes have been written on job interview techniques. The annotated bibliography lists some references.

The candidate should be asked to bring a resume to the interview. This provides an outline for discussing work history and training. Attitudes about mental health are of course important, but familiarity with office procedures is the criti-

cal element. More intelligent, well-read candidates have a vocabulary that makes dictation and transcription less cumbersome for all. While high intelligence can be an asset, it is only
one qualification for a satisfactory employee.

Part of the interview should be given to testing. Typing
speed can be validated. Spelling skills and depth of vocabulary can also be established by appropriate tests.

Hiring. No one should be hired on the spot. The therapist should have a chance to form an impression in the candidate's absence and should take time to check references.
However, if someone is obviously unsuited for the job, he
should promptly and diplomatically be informed that he is
not under consideration. One can inform possible candidates
that several people have applied for the job and a decision
will be rendered by a specific date. Often if a person is particularly enthusiastic about the job, he will write or call in the
interim.

References. References are absolutely critical. After all,
most behavioral scientists assert the best prediction of future
performance is past performance. Letters should be from recent employers and those in a position to evaluate the employee's performance. The therpist should try to call the reference. Few letters contain negative appraisals, but a candid
telephone conversation can be very informative.

Probationary Period. Office staff are frequently hired for a
probationary period of 14 to 90 days. During that time, the
employer determines the employee's fitness for the job. A
contract or an agreement may be drawn up specifying the responsibilities the job entails as well as the terms of the salary
and other benefits. The probationary period provides the
employer and employee an opportunity to sever the arrangement if necessary.

Hiring Professional Staff

Chapter 8 explored group practice. If and when the
therapist wishes to hire professional staff, the following
procedure is recommended.

Recruitment. Recruiting professional staff is different

than recruiting office staff. Informal methods, such as word of mouth, are often used. Because personality plays such an important role, other qualifications are sometimes unfortunately overlooked. Compatibility is almost as critical as professional qualifications, but a professional staff member should be qualified to practice in his own right. The following are the three major mental health disciplines with minimal qualifications of each for private practice and third-party reimbursement generally considered acceptable.

Social Worker
1. Master's degree in social work, and/or
2. Certification by Academy of Certified Social Workers, and/or
3. Certification or licensure as social worker in states where statutes exist.

Psychologist
1. Doctorate in psychology (Ph.D., Ed.D. or Psy.D.), and
2. Licensure or certification as psychologist, and
3. a. Certification by the American Board of Professional Psychology in Clinical, Counseling and/or School Psychology, or
    b. Listing by the National Register of Health Service Providers in Psychology.

Psychiatrist
1. Medical degree (M.D. or O.D.)
2. License as physician, and
3. a. Certification by the American Board of Examiners in Psychiatry and Neurology, or
    b. Eligibility for above certification.

There are many other mental health professionals not always licensed as independent mental health practitioners. These include master's degree counselors, psychiatric nurses, psychotherapists, and pastoral counselors. In some states these individuals are permitted to work in the private sector under supervision. In other states there is no restriction on individuals using these titles. Fully qualified, licensed practitioners are helpful in building a sound professional practice and image. Although license does not guarantee performance, it does mean that minimal requirements have been met.

If one cannot to recruit from personal resources, other efforts will have to be made. Employment agencies are of little value here, but advertising and school placement services can be useful.

Advertising. A classified advertisement can be placed in both newspapers and professional periodicals describing the job succinctly. The inclusion of the following information will help attract qualified candidates:

1. Name of employer
2. Description of position, job title, responsibilities involved, permanent or temporary, full or part time
3. Minimum qualifications including any restrictions based on regional factors
4. Salary range
5. Closing date for application and date position commences
6. Indication of whether interview expenses are to be fully paid
7. List of documents that should accompany letter of application, i.e., references
8. Name and address of person to whom application should be directed.

In national periodicals, addresses or box numbers rather than telephone numbers, should be listed. Some professional organizations that have recruitment services are listed in the Appendix.

Employment Services. All colleges have some kind of employment service for graduates. Many teaching hospitals have such services, sometimes run informally by directors of internship and residency programs. These will probably be helpful in recruiting psychologists since most states require one to two years postdoctoral experience prior to licensing.

The primary drawback of college placement services is that they mostly deal with recent graduates who are unlikely to have experience. If a therapist is situated near a university, however, a call or letter to various department heads may produce some candidates.

Contractual Arrangements. A contract is more important for professional staff than office staff. If that seems too formal, a letter can be composed designating job description, responsibilities and compensation. In an age when written contracts have been demonstrated to help married couples assess and maintain their relationships, mental health practitioners should be able to benefit from the same process. A contract will pay dividends by reducing ambiguity and disappointment due to poor communication.

Individual practitioners differ in their preferences of the terms of contracts, but usually agree the following items be delineated.

1. *Licensure and/or Certification.* The employee must hold and maintain the state licensure and/or certification in the appropriate field or specialty area (psychologist, marriage counselor, etc.).

2. *Professional Affiliation.* The employee will belong to appropriate professional organizations which monitor ethical conduct of their members.

3. *Continuing Education.* The employee will be responsible for receiving a specified number of continuing education credits.

4. *Salary.* The employer will pay the employee wages for services rendered. Either the employee is paid a fixed hourly wage for all services, or he is paid at varied rates for contingencies and services such as individual therapy, group therapy, hospital and other on site consultation, and report writing. Terms of benefits (if any) are specified, including insurance, profit sharing, retirement, days off and vacation.

5. *Duties.* The employee will be available to provide specific services, which may include therapy, consultation, supervision, coverage, report writing, and correspondence and public relations.

6. *Supervision.* The extent and nature of the supervision the employee must receive is specified along with a statement of fees that may be charged if the supervision is provided by the employer.

7. *Malpractice.* The extent and limits of malpractice insurance coverage provided by the employer is specified.

8. *Restrictions.* The employee agrees not to engage in independent private practice in the same geographic area (specified) in which he is employed. The employee also agrees not to engage in private practice (either on his own or under the employ of another) in the same geographic area for a specified period of time (usually two years) after employment is terminated. Work in a public facility is usually not restricted.

9. *Accommodations, Equipment and Services.* The employer may agree to provide any of the following items: office space, furniture, dictation equipment, secretarial services, answering services, telephone services.

10. *Termination.* Conditions under which employment may be terminated are specified. Usually employment may be terminated by mutual agreement or by 90 days notice.

11. *Duration of Contract.* Usually the contract is binding for twelve months.

SPECIAL PROBLEMS

Although the major mental health disciplines have much in common, each has special problems. Recognizing these problems and developing methods to deal with them may mean the difference between limited and expanded financial success.

Psychologists

The psychologist as an independent mental health practitioner is still not recognized by some insurance companies.

In the last five years, however, there has been substantial movement by third-party payers to cover psychologists' services. This movement is correlated with the trend toward providing coverage for mental health services in general.

As discussed in Chapter 1 the generic nature of their title is problematic for psychologists.

An academic or experimental psychologist may qualify for licensing in many states. Insurance companies rightfully assert that these individuals are unqualified for private practice and that the company is unable to differentiate between them and qualified clinicians. The American Board of Professional Psychology and the National Register of Health Service Providers in Psychology have assumed a central role in certifying psychologists who are qualified clinicians. Major insurance carriers, such as CHAMPUS, provide coverage for psychologists qualified by the National Register. In addition, the Association for the Advancement of Psychology (AAP) has been instrumental in developing a national lobby for psychologists. Membership in AAP is a good investment for any psychologist in private practice.

The matter of third-party payment cannot be lightly dismissed. It is natural for clients to seek the services of practitioners whose fees are covered by insurance. Practitioners who are not covered often have to reduce fees in order to remain competitive. Other practitioners affiliate with psychiatrists in order to receive coverage. For some, such affiliation is an admission that they are "unqualified to provide independent services. " In many states where freedom of choice legislation is not in effect, some insurance companies require physician supervision of the psychologist. Freedom of choice legislation permits patients to be reimbursed for the services of any licensed psychologist.

Psychologists argue that they are qualified and trained to provide independent services. Moreover, they assert that a medical degree does not qualify a physician to supervise mental health services. However, when insurance companies demand such supervision, psychologists must make appropriate arrangements if they wish their patients to be reimbursed. It is helpful for psychologists to have working relationships with a number of physicians since insurance companies look for physician referrals in evaluating the claim. Patients therefore may be asked to have their physicians call to set up a formal referral or sign a release so the psychologist can call to establish the referral. Despite the obvious drawbacks of this arrangement, it allows the psychologist to communicate with the physician, and that communication is often instrumental in promoting future referrals.

Hospital Affiliation. Psychologists historically have had a secondary role to psychiatrists regarding hospital affiliation. They do not usually enjoy full membership privileges entitling them to vote or admit patients. Hospitals argue that psychologists as nonmedical personnel, should not have a primary role on hospital staffs. In a complaint filed with the Federal Trade Commission, the Association for the Advancement of Psychology (AAP) has taken the Joint Commission of Accredidation of Hospitals (JCAH) to task on this issue.* Psychologists argued that exclusion from hospital staffs represents a restraint of trade. Even while the case was being heard, many practitioners began to see what was interpreted as a shift in JCAH regulations toward permitting greater participation by psychologists. Psychologists affiliated with teaching hospitals through university alliances, have found such restrictions very burdensome. However, for most psychologists, especially private practitioners, exclusion from full hospital privileges has only been a minor irritant. Psychologists in private practice should try to affiliate with hospitals in order to:

1. Establish contacts with physicians for better public relations,
2. Improve communications with physicians regarding mutual patients who are hospitalized,

*Federal Trade Commission memorandum supporting investigation of Joint Commission of Accreditations of Hospitals and American Medical Association; filed by Nicholson and Carter, attorneys for the Association for the Advancement of Psychology, July 12, 1976.

3. Provide input regarding better psychological care of the hospitalized.

Consultation. Many schools have begun to look toward psychologists for help in dealing with problem children. Many psychologists with a background in educational theory and child development become school consultants.

In recent years a number of federal and state regulations have been passed requiring schools to deliver psychological services. The major impetus for these regulations is Public Law 94-142, called the Education for All Handicapped Children Act of 1975. The regulations apply to the area of special education, and serve children diagnosed or suspected of having difficulties regarding emotional disturbance, retardation, learning disabilities, neurological problems and other problems that interfere with learning. The regulations often mandate that these children receive clinical services through the auspices of the school. In some states licensing as a psychologist is insufficient qualification, and in order to provide services to a school, certification through the department of education is required. However, many schools are now contracting with clinical psychologists to provide psychotherapy to students on and off school grounds. Inquiries may be made to superintendents of schools, directors of pupil personnel services, or directors of special education. In most cases, psychologists' services are provided by contract on a consulting rather than a salary basis. In the case of consultations, the psychologist is paid for specific units of work and he absorbs the costs of typing reports and providing test material.

Coverage for Medication. Psychologists must make provisions for those cases in which treatment requires medication or is enhanced by medication. For example, some practitioners believe that treating endogenous depression without medical intervention is a form of malpractice. Although the psychologist is not licensed to prescribe medication, he should be familiar with psychotropic drugs and their indications, contraindications, effects and side effects. Such knowledge will help the psychologist determine when medical intervention is indicated and enable him to assist in the observation of a patient who is receiving medication.

Many private practice psychologists have arrangements with physicians, usually psychiatrists, who provide consultation or services regarding the medical aspects of mental health care. The ideal arrangement for a psychologist is to have a psychiatrist who provides assessments and consultations solely for prescribing medication. However, not many psychiatrists wish to confine themselves to such a narrow role. It is important that a full understanding be reached between both professionals before the consultation referral is made. Usually, the consulting psychiatrist will see the patient periodically to assess the effect of medication, but he will depend heavily upon the psychologist's observations.

Some practitioners argue that transference issues become confused in such a relationship. However, if both practitioners communicate well with each other, and their roles are clearly defined to the patient, transference problems will be minimized.

Psychiatrists

Medication. The license to prescribe medication distinguishes the psychiatrist from other mental health professionals. Medical treatment increases the risk of malpractice charges. In addition to good medical practice and careful follow-ups, record keeping is also an important safeguard against such charges. All medication transactions should be recorded in the patient's chart and a copy of any prescription stapled to the chart.

Many psychiatrists have a standing arrangement with a medical laboratory to provide routine testing when drugs are prescribed that produce greater risk of side effects.

The previous section dealt with psychiatric consultation for medication. Such consultations may help the psychiatrist round out his practice and become better known. The increased rapport with psychologists may result in referrals for psychotherapy, especially for schizophrenic or severly depressed patients.

Image. The mental health field has undergone an image change in the last decade. However, psychiatry, more than psychology or social work, is frequently associated with the treatment of the severely mentally ill. A psychiatrist interested in couples therapy, school consultation or other areas associated with a "healthier" population, must make an extra effort to educate referral sources about his skills and interest. Probably the best ways of educating others are by conducting workshops, or giving talks that focus on his interests and skills. In time, the psychiatrist will become associated with the topics presented, and his image will be more consistent with the services he wishes to provide.

Social Workers

Many social workers in private practice complain about the impossibility of receiving third party payment. The move toward reimbursing social workers for services has been the slowest in the mental health field. The National Association for Social Work has been leading the attempt to educate insurance companies and legislators regarding the benefits of recognizing social workers as qualified independent practitioners. Meanwhile, social workers in private practice operate at a distinct disadvantage. Among the strategies frequently employed are entering into a formal relationship with a psychiatrist or psychologist who has greater access to third-party payment. If the relationship is carefully defined, the social worker may qualify for payment under the aegis of the other professional. However, some feel that such an arrangement further compromises the position of the social worker. Therefore, social workers more than other professionals, use sliding fees to compensate for the fact that their services are not covered by insurance.

Social workers, like psychologists, may also need to work out an arrangement with a physician or psychiatrist for medical treatment of certain disorders.

10 BENEFITS

Much of the clinician's time is spent assisting others improve the quality of their lives. But what can the mental health practitioner do to improve the quality of his own life? Although the independent practitioner has the opportunity to be self-directed, much of his energy is involved with income producing activities. While the employed clinician's choice of vacation time may be limited, the private practitioner may feel unable to take any vacation for fear of adverse economic consequences. Furthermore, private practitioners do not have the fringe benefits provided to employees at hospitals and other institutions. In addition to paid holidays and vacations, these benefits may include unemployment insurance, disability insurance, sick leave, health, dental and life insurance, and a retirement program. The independent practitioner must provide such benefits for himself.

This chapter deals with the benefits the practitioner can provide for himself, as well as strategies for acquiring those benefits without jeopardizing capital or financial fluidity.

INSURANCE

Before purchasing insurance one should know the kind and amount he needs. The term "insurance poor" is used to describe people who pay so much in insurance premiums that they don't have money enough to meet their present needs. In order to avoid being insurance poor but still be adequately covered, one must determine the financial risks he can afford to take.

There is no formula for deciding the kinds and amount of insurance to buy. The purchase of insurance may reflect a concrete plan of action or it may be a response to anxiety about the future. *The Consumers Union Report on Life Insurance* (Consumers Union, 1977) provides comprehensive information on this subject. Occasionally *Consumer Reports* magazine compares the cost and benefits of various insurance plans. The following kinds of insurance plans are typical of those purchased by practitioners.

Life Insurance

The two types of life insurance are term and equity. Term insurance, which is least expensive is collectable only in the event of death. Because it is relatively inexpensive, a young, healthy practitioner can purchase $50,000 or $100,000 of this type of insurance. Mortgages can also be covered by inexpensive term insurance policies.

Many professional organizations provide group rates for term insurance. However, these policies are sometimes only available to new members. Group rates are usually substantially lower than individual rates.

Equity or whole life insurance combines savings and life insurance. While a whole life policy pays the beneficiary less than a comparable term policy, it can be borrowed against or cashed in upon retirement. Frequently, practitioners buy both term and whole life insurance to provide protection as well as self-enforced savings.

The amount of insurance purchased should depend on

the premiums one can currently afford and the amount of money one's survivors would need. Other benefits they might receive, such as Social Security should be taken into consideration.

Disability and Sick Pay

There is no practical way for the self-employed therapist to provide sick pay benefits for himself in the way they would be provided at a clinic or hospital. However, disability insurance can protect the self-employed in the event of severe, long-term disability. The cost of the policy will be determined by the length of time one is willing to wait before receiving benefits and the amount of those benefits. A policy equivalent to sick pay benefits provided by clinics would eliminate any waiting period. Such policies are difficult to find, and, when they are available, are very expensive. Waiting periods are usually 30, 60, or 90 days. A policy with a 30-day waiting period usually carries a manageable premium. One should financially prepare for the waiting period by setting aside a sum of money equivalent to the benefits for that period of time. The benefits selected should be enough to sustain one's current standard of living, eliminating nonessentials.

A substantial portion of the disability payment will be tax free and the dollar value of the payments becomes greater than normal wages. In the case of total disability, Social Security may also be available.

Retirement Benefits

Under Individual Retirement Accounts (IRA) and the Keogh Plan (sometimes referred to as HR10), self-employed persons can set money aside in tax-free savings accounts or investment programs until retirement. For every dollar invested in the retirement fund, a dollar is substracted from gross income, thus reducing current tax liability.

The IRA has a lower investment ceiling than the Keogh

Plan and is usually utilized by employed individuals who do not have a retirement program available to them. The IRA is usually set up as a special savings account and is quite simple to arrange.

The Keogh plan is more complex. The money may be put into investments or insurance, but the investments must be executed by a disinterested party, such as a bank or insurance company, who complies with special federal regulations. Money placed in the Keogh Plan and in the IRA is available upon retirement at age 55 or older or upon disability or death. If money is withdrawn from the retirement program sooner, substantial financial penalties are imposed by the IRS.

The Keogh Plan also requires that after two years an employer covered by the plan must eventually provide employees with a similar plan, contributing to it the same percentage of their salaries as he does of his own. It would be beneficial to consult with an accountant or a tax attorney before investing in the Keogh Plan or an IRA.

Health Insurance

Hospitalization and related medical care are so expensive that few people can afford not to have health insurance. There are two types of health insurance. In the traditional kind policyholders pay an insurance premium and in the event of illness or hospitalization, go to the doctor or hospital of their choice. The insurance company provides reimbursement based on the terms of the contract purchased. An alternative form of insurance available in some cities is a health maintenance organization. Premiums support a specific group of doctors who provide the insured with in and outpatient services. These plans usually cost less than traditional plans but the patient is limited in his choice of doctors.

Group insurance rates are considerably lower than individual rates. A private practitioner may qualify for a group, for example through a part-time university job. A part-time employee may not be eligible to have the university pay for his insurance but he may qualify for the university's less expensive group rates. The same may be true for a practitioner who works as a part-time industrial consultant.

Although most health insurance policies cover some psychotherapy expense, some still do not. Before purchasing a policy, a therapist should determine what kind of mental health coverage it provides. He may not want to support a company that does not provide adequate coverage in his own field.

Malpractice Insurance

Malpractice or professional liability insurance is a work benefit invariably provided for clinic and hospital staff. The cost of such insurance is much lower for mental health practitioners than for most physicians. This fact reflects the relatively small number of successful claims against mental health professionals. However, the number of claims against mental health professionals has risen in recent years. Consequently, insurance rates have also risen. Malpractice insurance is a necessity for the private practitioner. Even if a private practitioner is incorporated, he can be held personally liable for damages claimed by a patient. A successful suit of $125,000 may result in bankruptcy for the uninsured. Even an unsuccessful suit may cost $10,000 in legal fees. Malpractice insurance provides for attorneys' fees and defense costs. Various liability limits are provided by insurance companies. Often, the cost of $1,000,000 coverage may not be much greater than $500,000.

Malpractice insurance for mental health professionals can be inexpensively purchased on a group basis through one of the major professional groups, such as the American Psychological Association, American Psychiatric Association or the National Association of Social Workers. Addresses are provided in the appendix.

135

VACATIONS AND DAYS OFF

In Chapter 1, it was suggested that income be projected on a 48 week, rather than 52-week basis. This is recommended so that vacation time can be incorporated into fiscal planning. Most industry provides a minimum of ten days off for holidays and at least one week a year for vacation. The importance of free time has been well established by industrial psychologists. Mental health practitioners sometimes fear that a vacation results not only in loss of current income but future income; that ambivalent patients may drop out of therapy; that new referrals will be lost. These concerns are not entirely unrealistic, but a practitioner whose life has become stultified by constant work may loose the drive necessary to maintain referral sources and keep up his business practices.

Lunch Hour

When one young psychologist began private practice, he spent noontimes at the Y, playing paddle ball and swimming a few laps. As his practice grew, he began to find it necessary to see patients during lunch hour. He began to feel less energetic and soon realized that he was giving up an important part of his life in order to increase the size of his practice. Finally he decided that, barring a legitimate emergency, the time between 12:00 and 1:00 was his alone. He found that the patients he'd seen during that hour were able to come in at other times.

The days of employees forced to work without lunch hours are long gone. The self-employed practitioner must be as reasonable an employer as he is a competent worker. It is as unhealthy for the employer to work without respite as it is for his employees.

Workshops

Workshops and continuing education programs present

a double expense—loss of the day's income and the cost of the program. This expense inhibits some practitioners from continuing their educations. However, many professional organizations and state licensing boards require continuing education for membership and license renewal. These requirements are imposed with good reason. The private practitioner, who works in isolation, has the sole responsibility for improving and maintaining his skills. Clinics and other facilities often provide formal or informal continuing education for their employees.

One way to learn about continuing education programs is to join or be placed on the mailing lists of professional associations that sponsor them. The appendix lists such professional organizations. In addition, many teaching hospitals regularly sponsor workshops or seminars and will mail announcements upon request. Another alternative is a study group in which practitioners meet on a monthly basis to share techniques, knowledge and ideas. Usually such groups are outgrowths of frequent professional contact. Although study groups do not always meet formal continuing education requirements, they tend to be stimulating and help keep the practitioner from becoming too isolated.

Continuing education should be regarded as an investment. New ideas and enthusiasm generated at workshops often provide the practitioner with both the incentive and the skills for building, maintaining and expanding his practice.

Coverage

Legally and clinically a practice must be covered when a therapist takes time off. Group practice members easily cover for each other, but single practitioners have more difficulty. If patients are suicidal, or in crisis, proper coverage is even more critical. For short vacations of one to three days, an answering service can be instructed to contact the therapist in any crisis. However, for longer vacations it is necessary for another practitioner to provide coverage. A colleague, preferably in the same discipline, may be willing to be contacted by patients in crisis in return for a similar favor at some point. The covering therapist should be given the names, important details, and instructions about any patient who is likely to call. If patients are given sufficient notice, and that notice is presented in a positive way, few problems usually arise.

The answering service should be instructed to tell callers the date and time the therapist is expected back. It should take name's and number's of individuals calling for appointments and should assure them that they will be called promptly when the therapist returns. This procedure will help alleviate the anxiety of patients who might be upset by the therapist's absence. Naturally, the answering service should be given the name and phone number of the covering practitioner.

REFERENCES

Consumers Union (Jan. 1978): "Are you paying too much for your phone?" *Consumer Reports,* 43: No. 1, pp. 50-53.

Council for the National Register of Health Service Providers in Psychology (1975): *National Register of Health Service Providers in Psychology,* Council for National Register of Health Service Providers in Psychology, ed. Baltimore, Maryland.

Fowler, D.R. (Winter 1976/77): "Current Practice in Psychiatric Utilization Review". *Int. J. Ment. Health,* 5: No.4, pp. 49-57.

Fowler, D.R. (June 1978): "The Psychiatrist and Health Insurance Claims Review". *J. Clin. Psychiatry,* 39: No. 6, pp. 519-522.

Fowler, D.R., and Longabaugh, R. (July 1975): "The Problem Oriented Record: Problem Definition". *Arch. Gen. Psych.,* 32, No. 7, pp. 831-834.

Fowler,D.R., Longabaugh, R., Sullivan C., Walker, M., and Nunez, N. (1977): "The Problem Oriented Psychiatric Team". *Int. J. Ment. Health,* 6: No. 2, pp. 17-25.

Grant, R.L., Maletzki, B. (1972): "Application of the Weed System to Psychiatric Records". *Psychiatr. Med.* , 3: pp. 119-129.

Joint Commission on Accreditation of Hospitals (1974): *Accreditation Manual for Psychiatric Facilities,* Joint Commission on Accreditation of Hospitals, ed. 2, Chicago, Illinois.

Lewin, M.H. (1978): *Establishing and Maintaining a Successful Professional Practice,* Rochester, New York, Professional Development Institute.

Longabaugh, R., Fowler, D.R., Sullivan, C., Walker, M., and Nunez, N. (1977):" The Problem Oriented Record in Quality Review, Program Planning, and Clinical Research". *Int. J. Ment. Health,* 6, No.2, pp. 76-88.

Ridgewood Financial Institute, Inc. (Feb. 1978): "Special Report: Fee and Practice Survey." *Psychotherapy Finances,* 5, No. 2, pp. 1–8.

Ryback, R. (1974): *"The Problem Oriented Record in Psychiatry and Mental Health Care,"* New York, Grune & Stratton Inc., p.4.

U.S. Dept. of the Treasury. Internal Revenue Service. Tax Guide for Small Business. (Pub. 334). Washington, D.C.: U.S. Government Printing Office.

Weed, L. (1970): *"Medical Records, Medical Education and Patient Care".* Cleveland, Ohio, Case Western Reserve University, pp. 154-161.

ANNOTATED BIBLIOGRAPHY

Private Practice Manuals

Lewin, Mark H. *Establishing and Maintaining a Successful Professional Practice.* Rochester, N.Y.: Professional Development Institute, 1978.

>One of the first private practice handbooks to be published. Originally priced at $25, this 177-page volume, privately published, may be purchased by writing to the Upstate Psychological Service Center, 765 Main St., Rochester, NY 14505. Although the book is oriented towards psychologists, it may have more universal appeal. A self-administered "Pre Private Practice Personality Profile" will be helpful to individuals wishing to explore their own compatibility with the stresses of private practice.

Shechtman, Morris. *Private Practice Manual.* Chicago: Center for the Study of Private Practice, 1977.

>Also a privately published work, rather brief (only 37 pages of text) and presented in outline form. This $16.50 manual may be purchased by writing to the publisher at the following address: Suite 3700, 75 East Wacker Drive, Chicago. Ill. 60601. The manual explores many problems of professional identity.

Private Practice as a Business

Psychotherapy Finances. South Orange, N.J.: Ridgewood Financial Institute.

    A monthly newsletter with a subscription price of $36/year, concerned with both professional and personal finances, such as fees, office expenses, taxes, and investments. A typical issue includes such titles as: "Is This the Year to Diversify Your Practice?"; "The Industrial Connection"; "Investing in Banks' Pooled Funds"; and "Will Sliding Fee Scales Cut Your Collections?". An advice column and notes of professional interest are also included in each issue.

Institute for Business Planning. *Closely Held Business.* Englewood Cliffs, N.J.: IBP.

    Written in non-technical language, this business service, with its twice-monthly supplements, provides complete and up-to-date coverage of all small business financial matters. Among the topics it considers are corporate formation and operation, pay packages, retirement plans, raising capital and accounting methods.

Kamaroff, Bernard. *Small Time Operator: How to Start Your Own Small Business, Keep Your Books, Pay Your Taxes, and Stay Out of Trouble.* Laytonville, Calif. Bell Springs Publications, 1976.

    The author, a financial advisor and tax accountant, while writing with a light hand, carefully and competently leads the reader through the maze of setting up and operating a small business. Although it is aimed at a retail operation rather than a professional office, it is an extremely helpful guide to the financing, technicalities and regulations of starting a business. There are also chapters on bookkeeping, becoming an employer, incorporating and taxes, as well as a complete set of ledgers.

Accounting

Ragan, Robert C. *Step by Step Bookkeeping.* New York: Drake, 1974.

    For the small businessman who does not have a full-time bookkeeper, this is a comprehensive guide to understanding what records to keep and how to keep them. It fulfills the promise of its title in that it is an excellent how-to text for someone who is inexperienced in bookkeeping procedures.

Taetzsch: Lyn and Taetzsch, Laura. *Practical Accounting for Small Businesses.* New York: Petrocelli/Charter, 1977.

This is a step-by-step guide to accounting procedures, but treated in greater depth than the above title. After an introduction to accounting theory, the authors explore the entire realm of accounting practices for small businesses. A chapter on preparing financial statements is especially helpful, as is a complete guide to payroll witholding and reporting obligations.

Taxes

P-H Doctor's Tax Report; Personal and Professional Tax Savings. Englewood Cliffs, N.J.: Prentice-Hall.

A bi-weekly newsletter provides up-to-date information about tax laws, rulings, and strategies. Subscription rate $120/year.

U.S. Dept. of the Treasury. Internal Revenue Service. *Tax Guide for Small Businesses. (Pub. 334).* Washington, D.C.: U.S. Government Printing Office.

This is a must-read for anyone setting up a practice in order to know what the IRS will expect from him at tax time. As stated in the introduction, it "is designed to answer the specific questions on Federal tax laws as they apply to business operations." Included is a summary of major changes in the tax law and a Tax Calendar/Check List which indicates what to do and when to do it. It is published annually, as is *Your Federal Income Tax (Pub. 17)*, another IRS publication which is helpful for filing your individual returns. Both may be obtained free from any IRS office.

Personal Finances

Blodgett, Richard E. *The New York Times Book of Money.* Rev. ed. New York: Quadrangle, 1976.

This book is a good basic introduction for the financial novice. Included are chapters on budgets, savings, loans, home ownership, insurance, educational expenses, medical care, taxes, retirement plans and investments.

Porter, Sylvia. *Sylvia Porter's Money Book; How to Earn It, Spend It, Save It, Invest It, Borrow It — and Use It to Better Your Life.* Garden City, N.Y.: Doubleday, 1975.

This is an all-round excellent source of personal financial information. A hefty 1105 pages long, it explores in depth all facets of the field. Part III, Managing Your Money, is especially helpful for financial planning; investments, pensions, social security, and life insurance are all discussed in detail.

Life Insurance

Belth, Joseph M. *Life Insurance: a Consumer's Handbook.* Bloomington, Ind.: Indiana University Press, 1973.

    Written by a professor of insurance in the School of Business at Indiana University, this book is very specific in its treatment of the subject. It presents information on the amount and type of life insurance to buy, and from whom to buy it. In addition, it discusses sources of insurance other than commercial insurance companies, e.g., banks and benefit societies. It also helps in explaining the fine print of an insurance policy.

Consumer Reports, eds. *The Consumers Union Report on Life Insurance: a Guide to Planning and Buying the Protection You Need.* Rev. ed. New York: Grossman, 1973.

    Another consumer-oriented publication, it covers much the same information as the above title. It stresses that it is important to determine how much life insurance is absolutely necessary. Excessive purchases are discouraged. There is also an extended discussion of social security as a type of insurance most people already have.

Investments

Engel, Louis. *How to Buy Stocks.* 6th rev. ed. Boston: Little, Brown, 1976.

    This is a classic in the field of investment books for the layman. Frequently revised to keep its information current, it provides the reader with a complete introduction to the investment market. It is especially helpful for its detailed description of the kinds of securities you may buy.

Soble, Ronald L. *Smart Money in Hard Times; a Guide to Inflation-Proof Investments.* New York: McGraw-Hill, 1975.

    Included here to illustrate the options available if the stock market makes you nervous, the book covers investments in gold and silver, gems, art works, coins, foreign currency, real estate, and bonds and short-term money market instruments. Not an in-depth treatment, but interesting reading if you are thinking about doing something different with your money.

U.S. News and World Report, eds. *How to Buy Real Estate: Profits and Pitfalls.* New York: Collier/Macmillan, 1970.

    The book is divided in two parts, the second of which deals with buying your own home. Part One is concerned with investing in real estate. The advantages as well as the disadvantages of investing in real estate are presented with additional discussion of what kind of real estate to buy, including commercial property and apartments. It is a good introduction to the options to consider if you are contemplating investing in real estate.

Clinical Records and Report Writing

Ryback, Ralph S. *The Problem Oriented Record in Psychiatry and Mental Health Care.* New York: Grune and Stratton, 1974.

    Recommended reading for anyone interested in the need for standardized documentation of mental health care records using the problem oriented approach. In this book, the author has taken the POR of Lawrence Weed for physicians and applied it to psychiatric care. He discusses the rationale for the POR and presents its application in several mental health care milieus. In addition, he considers the implications of the POR and computerization, and its use for professional standards reviews.

Tallent, Norman. *Psychological Report Writing.* Englewood Cliffs, N.J.: Prentice-Hall, 1976.

    A useful learning tool for writing psychological reports, it includes a discussion of the purpose of the report and what it should contain. Also considered are the organization of the report and how it can be used effectively. New concepts in psychological report writing are also discussed.

Consultation

Caplan, Gerald. *The Theory and Practice of Mental Health Consultation.* New York: Basic Books, 1970.

    After first defining mental health consultation, the author describes how practitioners can develop consultation programs in a community. He tells how to build a relationship with both the consultee institution and the consultee. He then presents various types of consultation with helpful advice for when taking on a consultant's role.

Kadushin, Alfred. *Consultation in Social Work.* New York: Columbia University Press, 1977.

In this book social work consultation is first defined and then described in detail. The essential steps in the consultation process are presented, from contact to termination, and the needs and attitudes of both parties in the process are considered.

Mannino, Fortune V., MacLellan, Beryce W., and Shore, Milton F., eds. *The Practice of Mental Health Consultation.* New York: Gardner Press, 1975.

This book discusses the practice of mental health consultation in a number of settings, e.g., with juvenile police, schools, and youth organizations. It describes the training of mental health consultants and explores some of the problems in consultation. Included is a guide to consultation literature, a helpful feature for anyone wishing to do more reading in this specific field.

Malpractice and Other Forensic Issues

Dawidoff, Donald J. *The Malpractice of Psychiatrists: Malpractice in Psychoanalysis, Psychotherapy and Psychiatry.* Springfield, Ill.: Charles C. Thomas, 1973.

Aimed at the psychiatrist, but extremely valuable for others in the mental health care field, this book discusses the tenets of malpractice, e.g., breach of duty, undue influence and words negligently spoken, and shows how they can be applied to the verbal therapies. This is a comprehensive treatment of a topic which is certainly of concern to all members of the mental health professions.

Sales, Bruce Dennis, ed. *Psychology in the Legal Process.* New York: Spectrum Publications, 1977.

A broadly-based review of forensic psychology, this book discusses numerous issues in the legal process and their psychological ramifications. Part III which deals with policy and professional issues has helpful chapters on the role of psychologists in child custody cases and the mental health professional as a witness.

Slovenko, Ralph. *Psychiatry and the Law..* Boston: Little, Brown, 1973.

The author is a law professor with a formal background in clinical psychiatry. Areas covered include the right to treatment, confidentiality, divorce and child custody, and psychiatric malpractice.

Interviewing Job Applicants

Hecht, Robert M., Aron, Joel E. , and Siegel, Morton D. *Interviewing Techniques for the Non-Personnel Executive.* New York: Personnel Testing Service, 1968.

Although its folksy approach might reduce its appeal to professionals, this is a helpful pamphlet for anyone who feels uncomfortable hiring for the first time. It covers preparing for and conducting the interview, provides productive questions to ask, and discusses interpretation of the application form and reference checks.

Rosenblatt, S. Bernard, Cheatham, T. Richard, and Watt, James T. *Communication in Business.* Englewood Cliffs, N.J.: Prentice-Hall, 1977.

A general text on business communication, it includes a chapter on interviewing — how to open the interview, types of questions to ask, and guidelines for participating in the interview. Especially helpful is a list of the questions which are considered taboo under the Equal Employment Opportunity Commission's guidelines.

Stewart, Charles J., and Cash, William B. *Interviewing: Principles and Practices.* Dubuque, Iowa: Wm. C. Brown, 1974.

A comprehensive text, it begins with a general introduction to interviewing followed by chapters on communication principles and practices and questions and their uses. Each type of interview is then considered. The chapter on employment interviews discusses the use of interviewing in the selection process and offers suggestions for conducting and participating in the interview including the beginning, the questioning and the closing.

APPENDIXES

1. Summary of State Licensing and Certification Regulations for Psychologists

Credit: Compiled and reprinted by permission of the Office of Professional Affairs, American Pychological Association, 1200 Seventeenth Street, N.W., Washington, D.C. 20036

State	(L)/(C)	Year of Original Approval	Coverage	Educational Requirement	Post Degree	Supervised	TOTAL EXP.	ABPP Accepted?	Examination Mandatory?	Continuing Education Req'r. (renw.)?	Renewal	Psych. Members	Public Members	Terms	"Grandfather" Deadline
Alabama	(L)*	1963	Practice of Psychologists	Doctorate	–	–	0	yes	yes	no	2 yrs.	5	–	5	10/1/65
Alaska	(L)	1967	Practice of Psychology:					yes	yes	no		3	0	3	1/1/68
			–Psychologist	Doctorate	1	1			yes		1 yr.				
			–Psychological Associate	Masters	1	3			yes		1 yr.				
Arizona	(C)*	1965	Psychologist	Doctorate	–	–	0	–	yes	no	1 yr.	5	0	8	–
Arkansas	(L)	1955	Psychologist	Doctorate	–	–	0	–	yes	no	1 yr.	5	0	5	7/1/57
			Psychological Examiner	Masters					yes		1 yr.				
California	(L)	1957	Psychologist	Doctorate	1	2	2	yes	yes	no	2 yrs.	5	3	4	8/20/70
	(C)	1969	Psychological Assistant				2		yes						
Colorado	(L)	1961	Psychology	Doctorate	2	2	2	yes	yes	yes	1 yr.	5	0	5	7/1/63
Connecticut	(L)	1945	Psychologist	Doctorate	–	1	1	yes	yes	no	1 yr.	5	0	5	6/24/69
Delaware	(L)	1962	Practice of Psychology	Doctorate	2	2	2	yes	yes	no	1 yr.	5	0	3	6/11/64
Dist. of Col.	(L)	1971	Practice of Psychology	Doctorate	2	–	2	yes	yes	no	1 yr.	5	0	3	4/8/72
Florida	(L)	1961	Practice of Psychology	Doctorate	1	2	2	–	yes	no	1 yr.	5	0	4	6/22/61
Georgia	(L)	1951	Pract. of Applied Psych.	Doctorate	–	1	1	yes	yes	no	2 yrs.	5	0	5	5/1/53
Hawaii	(L)	1967	Practice of Psychology	Doctorate	–	1	1	–	yes	no	2 yrs.	5	2	2	6/6/68
Idaho	(L)	1963	Practice of Psychology	Doctorate	–	–	2	–	yes	no	1 yr.	3	0	3	7/1/64
Illinois	(C)	1963	Psychologist in Private Practice	Doctorate	–	–	2	–	yes	no	2 yrs.	5	0	5	8/15/71
Indiana	(C)	1969	Practice	Doctorate	3	–	3	yes	yes	no	2 yrs.	5	0	3	7/1/72
			Psychologist	Doctorate	–	–	3	yes	yes	no	2 yrs.				12/31/69

149

State		Yr	License title	Degree							Exp.				1976
Iowa	(L)	1974	Practice of Psychology / Pract. of Associate Psychology (Indep.)	Doctorate	1	1	1	yes	yes	no	1 yr.	5	2	3	
Kansas	(C)	1967	Psychologist	Masters	–	2	5	–	yes	no	2 yrs.	7	0	3	7/1/69
Kentucky	(L)	1948	Practice of Psychology	Doctorate	1	2	2	–	no	no	3 yrs.	5	0	4	7/1/65
			Practice of Psychology (Certificand)	Doctorate	–	–	1	–	yes	no	3 yrs.				
Louisiana	(C)	1964	Psychologist	Masters (contin.)	2	2	2	yes	yes	no	1 yr.	5	0	3	7/1/66
Maine	(L)	1953	Psychologist	Doctorate	–	–	–	yes	yes	no	2 yrs.	5	1	5	10/1/68
			Psychologist Examiner	Masters	–	1	1	–	yes	no	2 yrs.				
Maryland	(C)	1957	Psychologist	Doctorate	1	1	2	yes	yes	yes	1 yr.	5	0	3	12/31/59
Massachusetts	(L)	1971	Psychologist	Doctorate	1	2	2	yes	yes	no	2 yrs.	5	0	5	12/31/73
Michigan	(C)	1959	Consulting Psychologist	Doctorate	4	1	5	yes	waiv.	no	1 yr.	7	0	–	8/1/61
			Psychologist / Psychologist Examiner or Technician	Doctorate	1	1	1	–	waiv.	no	1 yr.				
Minnesota	(L)	1973	Consulting Psychologist	Masters	–	1	1	–	waiv.	no	1 yr.	11	4	4	7/1/75
			Psychologist	Doctorate	2	–	2	yes	yes	no	2 yrs.				
Mississippi	(C)	1966	Psychologist	Masters	2	–	2	–	yes	no	2 yrs.	5	0	3	7/1/67
				Doctorate	1	1	1	yes	yes	no	1 yr.				
Missouri	(L)	1977	Psychologist	Doctorate	–	–	1	–	yes	no	2 yrs.	5	0	5	4/28/78
				Masters	–	–	3	–	yes	no	2 yrs.				
Montana	(L)	1971	Practice of Psychology	Doctorate	1	–	2	yes	yes	no	1 yr.	3	0	3	1/1/73
Nebraska	(L)	1967	Practice of Psychology	Doctorate	–	–	0	–	yes	no	1 yr.	5	0	5	1/1/71
Nevada	(L)	1963	Practice of Psychology	Doctorate	1	–	1	–	yes	yes	2 yrs.	5	0	4	7/1/64
New Hampshire	(C)	1957	Psychologist	Doctorate	1	2	2	yes	yes	no	1 yr.	3	0	3	7/1/59
			Associate Psychologist	Masters							1 yr.				
New Jersey	(L)	1966	Practice of Professional Psychological Services	Doctorate	1	2	2	yes	yes	no	2 yrs.	8	1	3	1/1/68
New Mexico	(C)	1963	Psychologist	Doctorate	2	–	2	yes	yes	yes	1 yr.	5	0	3	12/31/64
New York	(C)	1956	Psychologist	Doctorate	2	–	2	yes	yes	no	2 yrs.	11	0	5	7/1/59
North Carolina	(L)	1967	Practicing Psychologist	Doctorate	2	–	2	yes	yes	no	1 yr.	5	0	3	7/1/69
			Psychological Examiner	Masters	–	–	0	–	yes	no	1 yr.				
North Dakota	(L)	1967	Psychologist	Doctorate	–	–	0	yes	yes	no	1 yr.	5	0	3	7/1/68
Ohio	(L)	1972	Pract. of Psychology	Doctorate	–	2	4	yes	yes	no	2 yrs.	6	1	5	11/22/76
			Pract. of School Psych.	Masters	3	4	4	–	yes	no	2 yrs.				
Oklahoma	(L)	1965	Practice of Psychology	Doctorate	–	2	2	–	yes	no	1 yr.	5	0	3	6/28/66
Oregon	(L)	1973	Practice of Psychology	Doctorate	–	2	2	–	yes	no	1 yr.	7	2	3	1/1/74
			Psychologist Associate	Masters	–	3	–	–	yes	no	1 yr.				

State / Province	(L)/(C)	Year	Title	Degree							Term				Date
Pennsylvania	(L)	1972	Practice of Psychology	Doctorate	3	1	2	yes	yes	no	2 yrs.	7	0	3	5/23/72
				Masters	4	2	4	–	yes	no	2 yrs.				
Rhode Island	(C)	1969	Consulting Psychologist	Doctorate	1	2	2	yes	yes	no	1 yr.	3	0	3	12/31/70
			Academic Psychologist	Doctorate	1	2	2	yes	yes	no	1 yr.				
South Carolina	(L)	1968	Practice of Psychology	Doctorate	–	2	0	yes	waiv.	no	2 yrs.	7	0	5	3/21/69
South Dakota	(L)	1976	Psychologist	Doctorate	–	2	1	–	yes	no	2 yrs.	5	1	3	7/1/77
			Psychologist Associate	Masters	–	2	1	–	yes	no	2 yrs.				
Tennessee	(L)	1953	Psychologist	Doctorate	–	1	0	yes	yes	no	perm	5	0	5	7/1/55
			Psychological Examiner	Masters	1	1	2	–	waiv.	no	1 yr.				
Texas	(L)	1969	Psychologist	Doctorate	–	1	0	–	no	yes	1 yr.	6	0	6	12/31/70
			Psychological Associate	Masters	1	1	2	yes	yes	yes	1 yr.				
Utah	(L)	1959	Practice of Psychologist	Doctorate	2	2	3	yes	yes	yes	2 yrs.	5	0	5	12/31/62
Vermont	(L)	1976	Practicing Psychologist	Doctorate	3	3	4	yes	yes	no	2 yrs.	3	2	5	6/30/77
			Psychological Associate	Masters	2	2	2	n.a.	yes	no	–				
Virginia	(L)	1966	Clinical Psychologist	Doctorate	2	2	2	yes	yes	yes	2 yrs.	5	0	5	none
			Psychologist	Doctorate	4	2	4	yes	yes	no	2 yrs.				
		1976	School Psychologist	Masters	1	1	1	yes	yes	yes	1 yr.				
Washington	(L)	1955	Psychologist	Doctorate	1	1	1	yes	yes	no	2 yrs.	5	0	3	6/10/66
West Virginia	(L)	1970	Practice of Psychology	Doctorate	5	5	5	yes	yes	no	2 yrs.	5	0	3	11/12/70
Wisconsin	(L)	1969	Practice of Psychology	Doctorate	1	1	1	yes	yes	no	1 yr.	4	1	3	7/1/70
Wyoming	(C)	1965	Psychologist	Doctorate	–	1	0	yes	yes	no		5	0	3	12/31/65
Canada															
Alberta	(C)	1960	Psychologist	Masters	–	–	0	–	no	no		8	0	1	4/11/62
British Columbia															
Manitoba	(C)	1966	Psychologist	Doctorate	–	–	0	–	yes	–		7	0	2	12/31/72
New Brunswick	(C)	1967	Psychologist	Doctorate	–	–	1	–	yes	no		5	0	1	6/1/71
Nova Scotia–P.E.I.															
Ontario	(C)	1960	Psychologist	Doctorate	1	1	1	–	yes	no	perm	5	0	5	6/11/66
Quebec	(C)	1962	Psychologist	Doctorate	–	–	0	–	no	no		8	0	1	none
Saskatchewan	(C)	1962	Registered Psychologist	Doctorate	–	–	0	–	no	–		5	0	2	12/31/66

*Psychology Licensing (L) or Certification (C) Law Summary

NOTES

CHART EXPLANATIONS

Three headings appear under the word *Experience;* namely, "Post-Degree," "Supervised" and "Total." The "Total" years listed refers to the overall minimum experience requirement for licensure applicants, broken down into "Post-Degree" or "Supervised" subgroupings if required.

"ABPP" stands for the American Board of Professional Psychology. ABPP confers the diplomate upon individuals who have successfully passed the ABPP examinations for the four principal fields in professional psychology. Information about the ABPP examinations, which some boards (indicated on chart) accept in lieu of the regular licensure or certification examination, can be obtained from the APA Office of Professional Affairs.

Three headings appear under *Examining Board,* indicating the makeup of the licensing or examining board. Public members are non-psychologist members serving to provide public interest input for the certification or licensure process.

Grandfathering Deadline refers to the last date for which psychologists can apply to the Examining Board for a license or certificate without submitting themselves to the examination process provided that they have been practicing at the time of the enactment or implementation of the licensing or certificate statute.

Certification and Licensure Laws:

All fifty states and the District of Columbia have enacted laws regulating the practice of psychology. The laws are either certification laws or licensure laws: Certification laws limit the use of the title "psychologist," while licensing laws regulate the use of the title and also define the scope of those activities that constitute the practice of psychology.

Psychology has over the years followed a generic licensure and certification model, similar to physician licensure. This means that permits to engage in public practice do not refer to specialty training within one of the four principal areas of applied psychology, which are *clinical, counseling, industrial/organizational,* and *school psychology.* The APA Code of Ethical Practice and the ethical codes adopted as part of the licensing and certification process do, however, mandate that psychologists practice only within the scope of their expertise and training.

Note: Ordinarily, licenses or certificates are not required for psychologists in academic (teaching) or research settings. State Psychology Examining Boards will be able to identify those activities for which a license or certificate is required, however.

State Examining Boards:

State licensing and certification laws are administered by psychology examining boards. (Note: The APA is not in any way involved with the administration of the laws.) INDIVIDUALS INTERESTED IN APPLYING FOR LICENSURE AND CERTIFICATION SHOULD CONTACT THE PSYCHOLOGY BOARD IN THEIR STATE FOR COMPLETE AND UP-TO-DATE INFORMATION REGARDING THE REQUIREMENTS FOR PRACTICE. A list of state examining board secretaries is available from the APA Office of Professional Affairs.

Standards and Requirements for Certification and Licensure:

Most state laws set the *Doctorate* degree as the minimum requirement for licensure or certification as a psychologist, qualified for *independent* practice. The degree must be in a *field of study primarily psychological in nature*, as determined by the State Examining Board for Psychology. Most state laws also specify that the degree shall have been issued by an *accredited institution*. Additionally, degrees earned from a psychology program accredited by the American Psychological Association are held to be acceptable.

Some states certify those with Master's level training in professional psychology as *psychological assistants or associates*. The psychological assistant or associate functions under the supervision of a fully qualified (licensed or certified for independent practice) psychologist. At least one year of full time graduate study is needed to earn a Master's degree. An additional three to five years of graduate work and training is required in order to get a Ph.D. In clinical or counseling psychology, the requirements for the Ph.D. usually include an additional year of internship or supervised experience.

As to the testing procedures for licensure and certification, most state psychology examining boards require an examination, either written or oral. Many states employing a written examination use a standardized test developed by the Professional Examination Service.

Standards and Criteria for Practicing Psychologists:

The APA has developed a set of *Standards for Providers of Psychological Services*. The original *Standards* were approved by the APA Council of Representatives in 1974. A revised set of *Standards* limited to the four applied specialty areas were approved in January 1977. The *Standards* provide a minimum (or floor) level of achievement for practice. They are generic in the sense that they are applicable to all psychologists in practice. Specialty standards (for clinical, counseling, industrial-organizational, and school psychology) are being developed by a committee of the APA, however.

Psychologist Health Service Providers:

To provide consumers, third party payers, and government planners a clear idea of which generically licensed or certified psychologists are specially trained and qualified to render health services, the National Register for Health Service Providers in Psychology, an autonomous and independent organization, was established in 1975. Nearly 9,000 providers are listed in the most current edition of the *National Register*. In lieu of either national or state-by-state specialty licensure for health professionals, the Register assists the public in identifying qualified psychologist health professionals.

Peer Review: The State Psychological Association PSRC:

The APA has encouraged each state psychological association to set up a PSRC (Professional Standards Review Committee) to give consumers and third party payers an informal and readily accessible avenue of redress should a question arise as to the customary, usual and reasonable nature of any fee or service rendered. PSRC determinations are advisory in nature, and are based upon regional standards of practice as perceived by psychologist peers. Complaints about a practitioner that deal with more serious issues (for example, practice constituting a possible hazard to the public) can also be directed to the State Psychology Examining Board, the State Association Ethics Committee or to the American Psychological Association Committee on Scientific and Professional Ethics and Conduct.

153

2. Summary of State Licensing and Certification Regulations for Social Workers

Credit: Compiled and reprinted by permission of the National Association of Social Workers, Inc., 1425 H Street, N.W., Suite 600, Washington, D.C. 20005.

State	Year Passed	Type	Title	Education	Experience	Exam	Fees (Initial)	Fees (Renewal)	Exclusions (Public employees)	Exclusions (Private employees)	Exclusions (Students)	Privileged Communications	Reciprocity
Alabama	1977	L	Independent Practice	MSW	2	yes	Min	Min	yes	no	yes	no	yes
			Certified Social Worker	MSW	2	yes	$50	$25					
			Graduate Social Worker	MSW		yes							
			Bachelor Social Worker	BA	2	yes							
Arkansas	1975	R	Registered Social Worker	BSW	2	no	*	*	no	no	no	yes	no
			Registered Master Social Worker	MSW		yes							
California	1945	R	Registered Social Worker	MSW		no	$5–10	$3–11	yes	yes	no	yes	yes
				BSW	3	yes							
				BA	5	yes							
	1968	L	Licensed Clinical Social Worker	MSW		yes							
Colorado	1975	L	Licensed Social Worker(I)	MSW	2	yes	$50	$10	no	no	no	yes	yes
			Licensed Social Worker(II)	MSW	5	yes	$10–50	$2.50 –$20					
		R	Registered Social Worker	MSW	2	–							
				BA									
Delaware	1976	L	Licensed Clinical Social Worker	MSW	2	–							
Idaho	1976	L	Independent Practice	MSW	2	yes	*		yes	yes	no	yes	yes
			Certified Social Worker	MSW	2	no	$150		no	no	yes	yes	yes
			Social Worker	BSW		yes							
Illinois	1967	R	Certified Social Worker	MSW		yes	$25	$10	no	yes	yes	yes	yes
			Social Worker	BA	2	yes							

155

State	Year	L/R	Title	Degree	No.		Fee	Fee						
Kansas	1974	L	Independent Practice	MSW	2	yes	$10–50	$2.50–$20.	no	no	no	no	yes	yes
			"Specialties"	MSW	2	yes								
			Master Social Worker	MSW		yes								
			Bacc. Social Worker	BSW		yes								
			Social Work Associate	AA										
Kentucky	1974	L	Independent Practice	MSW	2	yes	Max $30	Max $30	yes	no	no	no	no	yes
			Certified Social Worker	MSW		yes								
			Social Worker	BSW		yes								
Louisiana	1972	L	Board Certified Social Worker	MSW		yes			yes	yes	yes	yes	yes	yes
Maine	1969	R	Registered Social Worker	MSW	2	yes	$50	$20	yes	yes	yes	yes	yes	yes
			Associate Social Worker	BA		yes	Max	Max						
Maryland	1975	L	Independent Practice	MSW	2	yes	$50	$10	yes	no	no	no	no	yes
			Certified Social Worker	MSW	2	yes	Max	Max						
			Graduate Social Worker	MSW	2	yes	$50	$50						
			Social Work Associate	BSW		yes								
Michigan	1972	R	Certified Social Worker	MSW	2	no	$25	$15	no	no	no	no	yes	yes
			Social Worker	MSW		no								
				BA	2	no								
			Social Worker Technician	2 yr.	1	no								
New York	1965	R	Certified Social Worker	MSW	2	yes	$40	$15	no	no	yes	no	yes	yes
Oklahoma	1965	R	Registered Social Worker	MSW	2	no	$5	$5	no	no	no	no	no	no
			Social Work Associate	BA	2	no								
Oregon	–1977	R	Registered Clinical Social Worker	MSW	2	no	Max $75	Max $50	yes	yes	yes	no	no	yes
			Social Worker	MSW		no	$3–5	$3–5						
Puerto Rico	1934	L	Social Worker	BSW	3	no			no	no	no	no	no	no
Rhode Island	1961	R	Registered Social Worker	MSW		no	$5	$1	no	no	no	no	no	no
South Carolina	1968	R	Registered Social Worker	MSW		no	$10	$5	no	no	no	no	no	yes
South Dakota	1975	L	Independent Practice	MSW		yes	*	*	no	no	yes	yes	yes	no
			Certified Social Worker	MSW		yes								
			Social Worker	BSW		yes								
			Social Work Associate	AA/BA		yes								

State	Year		Category	Degree		Fee						
Utah	1972	L	Independent Practice	MSW	2			no	no	no	no	yes
			Certified Social Worker	MSW	yes	$25						
			Social Service Worker	BSW	yes	$25						
			Social Service Aide		yes	$7.50						
Virginia	1966	L	Clinical Social Worker	MSW	yes	$60	$10	yes	yes	yes	no	yes
			Social Worker	MSW	yes							

Authority to set fees given to Board

157

3. Annotated List of the National Associations for Mental Health Practitioners*

AMERICAN ACADEMY OF CHILD PSYCHIATRY (AACP)
1800 R St., N.W., Suite 904   Phone: (202) 462-3754
Washington, DC 20009   Virginia Bausch, Exec. Dir
Founded: 1953. **Members:** 1700. Professional society of physicians who are in training or graduates of child psychiatry residency. To stimulate and advance medical contributions to the knowledge and treatment of psychiatric problems of children. Presents annual awards. Maintains 38 committees, including: Biologic Aspects of Child Psychiatry; Mental Retardation and Learning disabilities; Psychiatric Aspects of Infancy. **Publications:** (1) Newsletter, bimonthly; (2) Journal, quarterly; (3) Membership Directory, annual; also publishes monographs and newsletters.
Credit: See last page attached to annotated list

AMERICAN ASSOCIATION OF MARRIAGE AND FAMILY COUNSELORS (AAMFC)
225 Yale Ave.   Phone: (714) 621-4749
Claremont, CA 91711   Dr. C. Ray Fowler, Exec. Dir.
Founded: 1942. **Members:** 5000. **Staff:** 7. **Regional Groups:** 34. Professional society of marriage and family counselors. Assumes a major role in maintaining and extending the highest standards of excellence in this field. Has 12 accredited training centers throughout the U.S. and provides a nationwide marriage and family counseling referral service from its national office. Individuals serve as international affiliates in 13 foreign countries. **Publications:** (1) Journal, quarterly; (2) Newsletter, quarterly; (3) Membership Register, biennial. **Formerly:** (1970) American Association of Marriage Counselors.

*The list of organizations was derived from and reprinted by permission of *Encyclopedia of Associations*, Volume 1, Gale Research Company, Detroit, 1978, and the Reader's Service Bureau of the Gale Research Company. Organizations listed above were selected for reprint here where membership exceeded 1000 and the annotation indicated applicability to independent mental health practitioners. The listing here is not exhaustive, however. The reader is invited to explore Volume 1 for listings of smaller organizations as well as those that represent other interests. Volume 2 provides a listing of organizations by geographic area, and can be helpful to the reader wishing information about associations operating in his locality.

Appendixes

AMERICAN BOARD OF CLINICAL HYPNOSIS (ABCH)
C/O M. Erik Wright, Ph.D., M.D.
Depts. of Psychology & Psychiatry
University of Kansas   Phone: (913) 864-4131
Lawrence, KS 66045   M. Erik Wright, Ph.D., M.D., Coord.
Founded: 1958. Physicians, dentists, and psychologists. Certifying body for high-level accreditation of "expert" skills in using hypnosis in research and clinical practice. Sub-boards: American Board of Hypnosis in Dentistry; American Board of Medical Hypnosis; American Board of Psychological Hypnosis. Administers regional examinations periodically and board examinations annually.

AMERICAN BOARD OF PROFESSIONAL PSYCHOLOGY (ABPP)
C/O Dr. Margaret Ives
2025 I St., N.W., Suite 405   Phone: (202) 833-2730
Washington, DC 20006   Dr. Margaret Ives, Exec. Officer
Founded: 1947. Trustees: 12. **Staff:** 5. Certification board which conducts oral examinations and awards diplomas to advanced specialists in four professional specialties: Clinical Psychology, Industrial and Organizational Psychology, Counseling Psychology, and School Psychology. Candidates must have five years of qualifying experience in psychological practice. Presents Distinguished Professional Achievement Award annually. **Publications:** (1) Manual for Oral Examinations, annual; (2) Policies and Procedures, annual; (3) Directory of Diplomates, triennial. **Formerly:** (1968) American Board of Examiners in Professional Psychology.

AMERICAN BOARD OF PSYCHIATRY AND NEUROLOGY (ABPN)
1603 Orrington Ave., Suite 1320   Phone: (312) 864-0830
Evanston, IL 60201   Lester H. Rudy, Exec. Dir.
Founded: 1934. Diplomates: 12,898. Physicians with specialized training in psychiatry, neurology, or both. Determines eligibility requirements, administers examinations, and certifies physicians in the specialized fields of psychiatry and neurology.

AMERICAN GROUP PSYCHOTHERAPY ASSOCIATION (AGPA)
1995 Broadway, 14th Fl.   Phone: (212) 787-2618
New York, NY 10023   Marsha Block, Exec. Sec.
Founded: 1942. **Members:** 3000. **Staff:** 6. **Local Groups:** 22. Psychiatrists, psychologists, social workers and other mental health professionals who meet specific educational and professional requirements. Presents awards. Committees: Affiliate Societies; Audio-Visual Aids; Fellowship; History; Institute; International Aspects; Legislative Information; Liaison; Program; Research; Standards and Ethics. **Publications:** (1) International Journal of Group Psychothera-

160

py, quarterly; (2) Newsletter, semiannual; (3) Membership Directory, biennial; also publishes Consumer's Guide to Group Therapy, information about AGPA, brochure, brief history and guidelines.

AMERICAN NURSES' ASSOCIATION (ANA)

2420 Pershing Rd.   Phone: (816) 474-5720
Kansas City, MO 64108   Myrtle K. Aydellotte, Ph.D., exec.Dir.
Founded: 1896. **Members:** 200,000. **Staff:** 170. **State Groups:** 53. **Local groups:** 862. Professional organization of registered nurses. Sponsors American Nurses Foundation (research in nursing). Offers Pearl McIver Public Health Award for outstanding contribution to public health nursing; Mary Mahoney Award for significant contribution toward opening opportunities in nursing to minority groups. Maintains hall of fame and library. **Commissions:** Economic and General Welfare; Human Rights; Nursing Education; Nursing Research; Nursing Services. **Committees:** Ethics; Intergroup Relations. **Councils:** Adult and Family Nurse Practitioners and Clinicians; Advanced Practitioners in Medical-Surgical Nursing; Advanced Practitioners in Psychiatric and Mental Health Nursing; Advisory; Continuing Education; Nurse Researchers; Nursing Service Facilitators; Pediatric Nurse Practitioners; State Boards of Nursing. **Divisions:** Community Health; Geriatric; Maternal and Child Health; Medical-Surgical; Psychiatric and Mental Health Nursing. **Publications:** (1) American Journal of Nursing, monthly; (2) The American Nurse, monthly; (3) Capital Commentary, monthly; (4) Facts About Nursing, annual; (5) Biennial Reports to House of Delegates; (6) Proceedings of the House of Delegates, biennial; also publishes book. **Affiliated with:** International Council of Nurses. **Formerly:** (1911) Nurses Associated Alumnae of United States and Canada.

AMERICAN PERSONNEL AND GUIDANCE ASSOCIATION (APGA)

1607 New Hampshire Ave., N.W.   Phone: (202) 483-4633
Washington, DC 20009   Charles L. Lewis, Exec. V. Pres.
Founded: 1952. **Members:** 41,000. **Staff:** 50. **State Groups:** 51. Professional society of guidance and personnel workers in elementary and secondary schools, in higher education, in community agencies and organizations, government, industry, and business. Maintains special library (5000 books and pamphlets). Maintains placement service for members. **Committees:** APGA Insurance Trust; Commission on Human Rights; Ethical Practices; Federal Relations; International Education; Placement Service Review; Professional Preparation and Standards; Research Awards. **Divisions:** American College Personnel Association (ACPA); American Rehabilitation Counseling Association (ARCA); American School Counselor Association (ASCA); Association for Counselor Education and Supervision (ACES); Association for Humanistic Education and Development (AHEAD); Association for Measurement and Evaluation in Guidance (AMEG); Association for Non-White Concerns in Personnel and Guidance (ANWC); Association for Specialists in Group Work (ASGW); National Catholic Guidance Conference (NCGC); National Employment Counselors Association (NECA); National Vocational Guidance Association (NVGA); Public Offender Counselor Association (POCA). **Publications:** (1)

161

Guidepost (newsletter), 18/year; (2) Personnel and Guidance Journal, 10/ year; (3) Journal of College Student Personnel, bimonthly; (4) School Counselor, 5/year; (5) Counseling and Values, quarterly; (6) Counselor Education and Supervision, quarterly; (7) Journal of ANWC, quarterly; (8) Journal of Employment Counseling, quarterly; (9) Measurement and Evaluation in Guidance, quarterly; (10) Rehabilitation Counseling Bulletin, quarterly; (11) The Humanist Educator, quarterly; (12) Vocational Guidance, quarterly.

AMERICAN PSYCHIATRIC ASSOCIATON (APA)

1700 - 18th St., N.W.   Phone: (202) 797-4900
Washington, DC 20009   Melvin Sabshin, M.D., Med. Dir.
Founded: 1844. **Members:** 23,600. **Staff:** 100. **Regional Groups:** 71. Professional society of psychiatrists who have M.D. degrees. To further the study of the nature, treatment, and prevention of mental disorders. Assists states in formulating programs to meet mental health needs; develops standards for psychiatric facilities; compiles and disseminates facts and figures about psychiatry; furthers psychiatric education and research; maintains library. **Councils:** Children, Adolescents and Their Families; Emerging Issues; Internal Organization; International Affairs; Medical Education and Career Development; Mental Health Services; National Affairs; Professions and Associations; Research and Development. **Publications** (1) Psychiatric News, semimonthly; (2) American Journal of Psychiatry, monthly; (3) Hospital and Community Psychiatry, monthly; (4) Membership Directory; also publishes books and pamphlets. **Formerly:** (1892) Association of Medical Superintendents of American Institutions for Insane; (1921) American Medico-Psychological Association.

AMERICAN PSYCHOANALYTIC ASSOCIATION (APsaA)

One E. 57th St.   Phone: (212) 752-0450
New York, NY 10022   Helen Fischer, Adm. Dir.
Founded: 1911. **Members:** 2485. **Staff:** 10. **Local Groups:** 34. Professional association of medically oriented psychoanalysts who have graduated from an accredited institute. To establish and maintain standards for the training of psychoanalysts and for the practice of psychoanalysis; to foster the integration of psychoanalysis with other branches of medicine and to encourage research. **Publications:** (1) Journal of the APsaA, quarterly; (2) Newsletter, quarterly; (3) Roster, annual; also publishes Glossary of Psychoanalytic Terms and Concepts.

AMERICAN PSYCHOLOGICAL ASSOCIATION (APA)

1200 17th St., N.W.   Phone: (202) 833-7600
Washington, DC 20036   Dr. Charles Kiesler, Exec. Officer
Founded: 1892. **Members:** 45,000. **Staff:** 170. **State Groups:** 53. Scientific and professional society of psychologists and educators. Students participate as Student in Psychology subscribers. To advance psychology as a science, a

profession, and as a means of promoting human welfare. Boards: Convention Affairs; Education and Training; Policy and Planning; Professional Affairs; Publications and Communications; Scientific Affairs; Social and Ethical Responsibility. **Divisions:** Adult Development and Aging; Clinical Psychology; Community Psychology; Consulting Psychology; Consumer Psychology; Counseling Psychology; Developmental Psychology; Educational Psychology; Evaluation and Measurement; Experimental Analysis of Behavior; Experimental Psychology; General Psychology; History of Psychology; Humanistic Psychology; Hypnosis; Industrial and Organizational Psychology; Mental Retardation; Military Psychology; Personality and Social Psychology; Philosophical Psychology; Physiological and Comparative Psychology; Population Psychology; Psychologists Interested in Religious Issues; Psychologists in Public Service; Psychology and the Arts; Psychology of Women; Psychopharmacology; Psychotherapy; Rehabilitation Psychology; School Psychology; Society of Engineering Psychologists; Society for the Psychological Study of Social Issues; State Psychological Association Affairs; Teaching of Psychology. **Publications:** (1) American Psychologist, monthly; (2) Contemporary Psychology, monthly; (3) Employment Bulletin, monthly; (4) Journal of Personality and Social Psychology, monthly; (5) Monitor (newspaper), monthly; (6) Psychological Abstracts, monthly; (7) Developmental Psychology, bimonthly; (8) Journal of Abnormal Psychology, bimonthly; (9) Journal of applied Psychology, bimonthly; (10) Journal of Comparative and Physiological Psychology, bimonthly; (11) Journal of Consulting and Clinical Psychology, bimonthly; (12) Journal of Counseling Psychology, bimonthly; (13) Journal of Educational Psychology, bimonthly; (14) Journal of Experimental Psychology: Human Learning and Memory, bimonthly; (15) Psychological Review, bimonthly; (16) Psychological Bulletins, bimonthly; (17) Journal of Experimental Psychology: Animal Behavior Process, quarterly; (18) Journal of Experimental Psychology: General, quarterly; (19) Journal of Experimental Psychology: Human Perception and Performance, quarterly; (20) Journal Supplement Abstract Service, quarterly; (21) Professional Psychology, quarterly; also publishes Biographical Directory and Membership Register. **Affiliated with:** Psi Chi, the national honorary society in psychology. **Absorbed:** Psychologists Interested in the Advancement of Psychotherapy; (1976) Psychologists Interested in Religious Issues.

AMERICAN ORTHOPSYCHIATRIC ASSOCIATION (AOA)
1775 Broadway   Phone: (212) 586-5690
New York, NY 10019   Marion F. Langer, Ph.D., Exec. Dir.
Founded: 1924. **Members:** 4800. **Staff:** 14. Psychiatrists, psychologists, psychiatric social workers, and members drawn from related fields of anthropology, sociology, education, nursing and allied professions. To unite and provide a common meeting ground for those engaged in the study and treatment of problems of human behavior. To foster research and spread information concerning scientific work in the field of human behavior, including all forms of abnormal behavior. Maintains Public Issues Council. Study Groups: After-Care; Aggression and Violence; Aging; Anti-Racism Coordinating Group; Confidentiality of Health and Social Service Records; Cultural Pluralism; Mental Health in Schools; Native Americans; Professional Standards Review Organization; Women. **Publications:** (1) American Journal of Orthopsychiatry, 4/year; (2) Newsletter, semiannual; (3) Membership Directory; also publishes monographs.

Appendixes

AMERICAN SOCIETY FOR ADOLESCENT PSYCHIATRY (ASAP)
24 Green Valley Rd.   Phone: (215) 566-1054
Wallingford, PA 19086   Mary Staples, Exec.Sec.
Founded: 1967. **Members:** 1600. **Staff:** 1. **Local Groups:** 18. Qualified psychiatrists who are interested in adolescents. Conducts workshops at annual scientific meetings. Consults with national organizations interested in the welfare of youth. Bestows awards; holds occasional symposia on topics relating to adolescent psychiatry. **Publications:** (1) Newsletter, quarterly; (2) Annals of Adolescent Psychiatry, annual; (3) Membership Directory, biennial.

ASSOCIATION FOR ADVANCEMENT OF BEHAVIOR THERAPY (AABT)
420 Lexington Ave.   Phone: (212) 682-0065
New York, NY 10017   Elizabeth Ann Kovacs, Exec.Dir.
Founded: 1966. **Members:** 2200. Foreign and State Groups: 20. Psychiatrists and psychologists; about 5 percent of membership is social workers, dentists, medical engineers, physiotherapists, and other professionals interested in the issues, problems, and development of the general field of behavior modification, with specific emphasis on the clinical applications. Plans to develop training program and lectures for professionals and semi-professionals, organize a speaker's bureau, and arrange for communication between behavior therapists interested in specific problems or information. AABT branches hold training meetings, workshops, seminars, case demonstrations, and discussion groups. **Publications:** (1) Behavior Therapy Journal, 5/year; (2) Newsletter, bimonthly; (3) Membership Directory, annual. **Formerly:** (1968) Association for Advancement of the Behavioral Therapies.

ASSOCIATION FOR ADVANCEMENT OF PSYCHOLOGY (AAP)
1200 17th St., N.W., Suite 400   Phone: (202) 659-3888
Washington, DC 20036   Clarence J. Martin, Exec. Dir.
Founded: 1974. **Members:** 6000. **Staff:** 7. Members of the American Psychological Association or other national psychological associations, students of psychology, and organizations primarily psychological in nature. Purposes are to advance psychology and to represent the interests of all psychologists (professional, social and scientific) in the public policy arena. **Publications:** Advance (newsletter), monthly. **Affiliated with:** American Psychological Association.

ASSOCIATION FOR HUMANISTIC PSYCHOLOGY (AHP)
325 Ninth St.   Phone: (415) 626-2375
San Francisco, CA 94103   Elizabeth Campbell, Exec. Officer
Founded: 1962. **Members:** 6000. **Local Groups:** 50. Membership consists of

164

psychologists, social workers, clergy, educators, psychiatrists, laypeople. World-wide network for the development of human sciences in ways which recognize distinctively human qualities and which work toward fulfilling the innate capacities of people - individually and in society. Aims are "to link, support and stimulate people who have a humanistic vision of the person; to encourage others to share this view; and to show how this vision can be realized in the life and work of all." **Publications:** (1) Newsletter, monthly; (2) Journal, quarterly; (3) Dawnpoint Subscription Magazine, semiannual; also publishes Roster and other materials. **Formerly:** (1969) American Association for Humanistic Psychology.

AMERICAN SOCIETY OF CLINICAL HYPNOSIS (ASCH)

2400 E.Devon Ave., Suite 218   Phone: (312) 297-3317
Des Plaines, IL 60018   William F. Hoffman, Jr., Exec.Dir.

Founded: 1957. **Members:** 2600. **Staff:** 4. **State Groups:** 9. **Local Groups:** 31. Physicians, dentists, and psychologists with a doctoral degree. Brings together professional people in medical, dental, and psychological fields using hypnosis; sets up standards of training; conducts teaching sessions and workshops at basic and advanced levels. Through its affiliate, ASCH-Education and Research Foundation, offers periodic instruction on clinical hypnosis, various simple forms of psychotherapy, and psychodynamics. Sponsors legislative activity to help curtail use of hypnosis by entertainers. Cooperates with all scientific disciplines in professional and public relationships in regard to use of hypnosis. **Publications:** (1) News Letter, 8/year; (2) American Journal of Clinical Hypnosis, quarterly; (3) Directory (supplement to Journal), annual.

ASSOCIATION FOR WOMEN IN PSYCHOLOGY (AWP)

Dept. Of Psychology
Southern Illinois University   Phone: (618) 453-2374
Carbondale, IL 62901   Joyce Walstedt, Corres.Sec.

Founded: 1969. **Members:** 1200. Objectives are: to end the role which psychology has had in perpetuating unscientific and unquestioned assumptions about the "natures" of women and men; to encourage unbiased psychological research on sex differences, in order to establish facts and explode myths; to encourage research and theory directed toward alternative sex-roles, child raising practices, life-styles, and vocabularies; to educate and sensitize the psychology profession and the public to the psychological, social, political and economic problems of women; to achieve equality of opportunity for women and men within the profession of psychology. Holds "rap sessions" at annual meetings of American Psychological Association and of regional psychology associations. Maintains archives; bestows annual research award. Provides feminist therapists roster; sex discrimination complaint coordinator; feminist research notes. Monitors sexism in American Psychological Association. **Committees:** Speaker's Bureau. **Publications:** Newsletter, bimonthly; also publishes Feminist Internship Roster and Feminist Therapist Roster. **Formerly:** (1970) Association for Women Psychologists.

Appendixes

ASSOCIATION OF EXISTENTIAL PSYCHOLOGY AND PSYCHIATRY
C/O Dr. Louis De Rosis
40 E. 89th St.   Phone: (212) 348-3500
New York, NY 10028   Dr. Louis De Rosis, Sec.
Founded: 1960. **Members:** 1700. **Staff:** 3. Psychiatrists, psychologists, social workers, sociologists, theologians, teachers, college and university professors, philosophers, and others interested in a "multi-dimensional dialogue among all the disciplines which further the non-technological aspects of human existence." Sponsors public lectures, a seminar, and study groups. **Publications:** Review of Existential Psychology and Psychiatry, 3/year.

COUNCIL FOR THE ADVANCEMENT OF THE PSYCHOLOGICAL PROFESSIONS AND SCIENCES (CAPPS)
1200 17th St., N.W., Suite 400   Phone: (202) 466-8762
Washington, DC 20036   Jack Donahue, Exec. Dir.
Founded: 1971. **Members:** 3000. **Staff:** 3. State representatives: 51. Psychologists (private practitioners, clinicians, educators, researchers, counselors and industrial, military and public service psychologists). Purposes are: to educate Congress to the contribution psychology can make to the public; to educate psychologists to the legislative issues; to work toward increased governmental support in the education, training, and utilization of psychological manpower; to establish psychology's identity with the general public; to address issues where psychology's expertise can enlighten. **Committees:** Governmental Relations; Internship; Public Policy Research. **Publications:** (1) Keyperson Bulletin, monthly; (2) CAPPSule (newsletter), 12/year; (3) Washington Alert, irregular.

INTERNATIONAL TRANSACTIONAL ANALYSIS ASSOCIATION (ITAA)
1772 Vallejo St.   Phone: (415) 885-5992
San Francisco, CA 94123   Robert F. Anderson, Exec. Dir.
Founded: 1958. **Members:** 11,000. **Staff:** 17. A non-profit educational corporation of persons in medical and behavioral sciences, including psychiatrists, psychologists, social workers, nurses, teachers, probation officers, ministers, and physicians. ITAA is responsible for the standards of practice and teaching of transactional analysis, which is oriented toward group therapy, social dynamics, and personality theory based on analysis of the "transactions" or interactions between persons. The popular book, "Games People Play" covers basic transactional analysis theory; its author, Dr. Eric Berne, was ITAA founder. Grants Eric Berne Memorial Scientific Award annually. Maintains library of 1500 volumes on transactional analysis and related psychiatric works. **Publications:** (1) Script (newsletter), bimonthly; (2) Transactional Analysis Journal, quarterly; (3) Geographical List of Members, Subject and Name Indexes, annual. **Formerly:** (1961) San Francisco Social Psychiatry Seminar.

166

NATIONAL ASSOCIATION OF SOCIAL WORKERS (NASW)
1425 H St., N.W., Suite 600   Phone: (202) 628-6800
Washington, DC 20005   Chauncey Alexander, Exec.Dir.
Founded: 1955. **Members:** 75,000. **Staff:** 85. **State Groups:** 55. Regular members are persons who hold a minimum of a baccalaureate degree in social work. Associate members are persons engaged in social work who have a baccalaureate degree in another field. Student members are persons enrolled in accredited (by the Council on Social Work Education) graduate or undergraduate social work programs. Purpose is to promote the quality and effectiveness of social work practice by: advancing sound social policies and programs and utilizing the professional knowledge and skills of social work to "alleviate sources of deprivation, distress and strain"; setting professional standards; conducting study and research; improving professional education; publication and interpretation to the community. Maintains a library of 4000 volumes. Presents National Public Citizen of the Year and National Social Worker of the Year awards. Administrative Units: Academy of Certified Social Workers; NASW - Social Work Vocational Bureau; Publications Editorial Office. **Publications:** (1) Advocate for Human Services, biweekly; (2) NASW News, monthly; (3) Social Work, bimonthly; (4) Health and Social Work, quarterly; (5) Social Work Research and Abstracts, quarterly; also publishes Encyclopedia of Social Work, Directory of Professional Social Workers, Register of Clinical Social Workers and various books and pamphlets. **Formed by Merger of:** American Association of Group Workers; American Association of Medical Social Workers; American Association of Psychiatric Social Workers; American Association of Social Workers; Association for the Study of Community Organization; National Association of School Social Workers; Social Work Research Group.

SOCIETY FOR CLINICAL AND EXPERIMENTAL HYPNOSIS (SCEH)
205 West End Ave.   Phone: (212) 873-7200
New York, NY 10023   Marion Kenn, Adm.Sec.
Founded: 1949. **Members:** 750. **Local Groups:** 7. Professional society of physicians, dentists, psychologists and allied professional persons interested in research in hypnosis and its boundary areas as well as the therapeutic use of hypnosis in clinical practice. Encourages cooperation among professional and scientific disciplines in use of hypnosis, promotes educational standards, conducts introductory and advanced workshops. Gives several annual awards in recognition of outstanding contributions in the field of clinical and experimental hypnosis. **Publications:** (1) International Journal of Clinical and Experimental Hypnosis, quarterly; (2) Membership Directory, biennial; (3) Newsletter. **Affiliated with:** American Association for the Advancement of Science: World Federation of Mental Health.

4. Examples of Office Layout and Traffic Flow

Figure 1

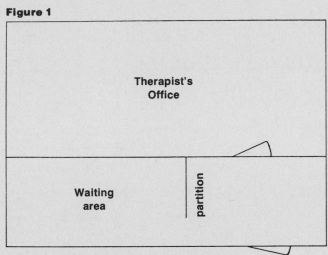

Figure 1 is for the solo practitioner who does not use a receptionist. Traffic is directed to maximize patient privacy.

Figure 2

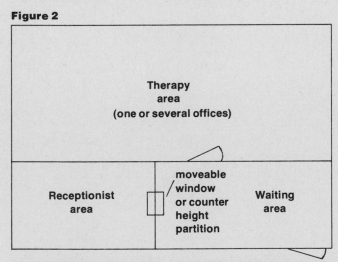

Figure 2 is designed to maximize patient exposure to the receptionist who may collect fees.

*The figures presented above are but a scant sampling of the many options available to the therapist. Office arrangements will vary according to type of therapy conducted and the physical limitations of the room.

Figure 3

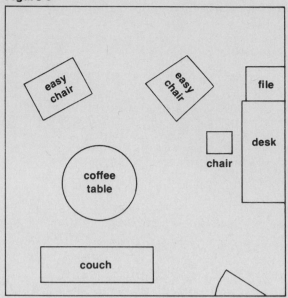

Figure 3 maximizes utilization of space in a small office (as small as 10′ x 10′).

Figure 4

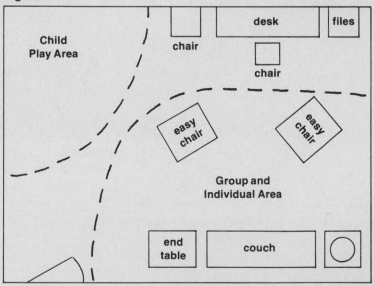

Figure 4 demonstrates how a larger area may be used to serve multiple purposes.

5. Release of Information Forms

Example of Two Way Release[1]

RELEASE OF INFORMATION [2]

I hereby authorize Dr. Allen G. Sheffield and _____ to release to each other any and/or all medical, psychological, or educational information they may have pertaining to _____ .

Signature _____ Date_____

Witness _____ Date_____

Example of One Way Release

RELEASE OF INFORMATION

I hereby authorize _____ to release to _____ any and/or all medical, psychological, or educational information pertaining to _____ .

Signature_____ Date_____

Witness _____ Date_____

[1]Two way forms are used to reduce the need for repetitive signing.

[2] Most printers will print up forms and bind them into convenience pads of 50 sheets each. Carbon paper may be used to produce copies so that signed forms do not have to be photocopied. The copies may be used for office reference, but may have limited legal value.

6. Report Form

REPORT FORM

BARBARA STEVENS-MUNCEY
PSYCHOLOGICAL SERVICES
1030 PRESIDENT AVE.
FALL RIVER, ILLINOIS 60614
TELEPHONE 673-8831

RE: _____ AGE _____

DATE _____

DEAR DR. _____

THANK YOU FOR REFERRING YOUR PATIENT. THE FOLLOWING IS A SUMMARY OF ESSENTIAL FINDINGS.

HISTORY: _____
_____
_____
_____
_____
_____
_____
_____
_____

DIAGNOSTIC IMPRESSION: _____
_____
_____
_____
_____

TREATMENT OR DISPOSITION: _____
_____
_____
_____

REMARKS: _____
_____
_____

SIGNED _____

173

7. Data Based Clinical Record Initial Evaluation and Treatment Plan

Patient:	R.F.J.
Birthdate:	3/31/31
Referred by:	Dr. Jonas Smith
	Medical Arts Clinic

Current Situation

The patient is a 46-year-old married man, referred by his physician for evaluation of depression. Patient states that he has felt "depressed for the past two months." (See problem # 1.) He has noted no weight loss, no decreased libido, no feelings of hopelessness. He denies suicidal thoughts. Onset of these symptoms corresponds to the time he was passed over for promotion for a younger man, whom the patient felt was "too aggressive." (See problem # 2.) In addition, shortly thereafter, his wife went to another state to care for her sick mother for two weeks. (See problem # 3.) Patient denies alcohol or drug abuse. Has 1 or 2 drinks only at parties.

Relevant Past History

Patient raised in this state. Father was a laborer. "He worked hard to put us through school." Died of a heart attack at age 54, immediately after patient, age 22, graduated from college (B.A. in business administration). Patient took job with insurance company, where he has worked since, rather than wait for a better job, because he felt obligated to support his mother.

Father worked two jobs to support family, and patient feels this contributed to his death. "He sacrificed for us." "I'll never be the man he was." (See problem # 5). Never felt emotionally close to father. Mother died four years ago at age 72 of a stroke. Patient shows sadness and cries when speaking of her death. "She worked hard too, bringing us up. She was the one we could bring our problems to."

Patient's only sibling, a brother 50 years old, is vice-president of a chemical manufacturing corporation. "He was always the go-getter in the family. He is not the kind anyone can get close to. He's his own man." Patient and brother have had little contact since the death of their mother.

There is no family history of depression or other emotional disorders.

Current Functioning

   Job: (See problem # 2.)

   Marriage: (See problem # 3.)

   Social Relationships - Leisure Time: (See problem # 4).

Physical Health

Report from Dr. Smith says patient is in good physical health. No evidence of organic disease to account for symptoms.

Mental Status

Looks his age. Wears tie and sport jacket. Slumps in chair. Appears anxious. States that he feels depressed. Cries briefly several times during the interview, but quickly changes subject. Shows deference to examiner. Thought content in keeping with depressed mood ("lack of enjoyment", "don't feel like it"). Has good memory for dates and times, and therefore no formal evaluation of sensorium and calculation ability was performed. Made no loose associations or bizarre statements. Shows some insight in recognizing that his feelings of depression are related to his job and recent events in his marriage, although he is not clear of the relationship.

The problems identified are listed in the following problem list.

Signed: _____
John Frazer, M.D.

PROBLEM LIST

Patient: R.F.J.

No.	Problem List	Date Activated	Date Resolved
1.	Feels depressed.	1/16/78	7/27/78
2.	Dissatisfied with job performance.	1/16/78	5/18/78
3.	Doesn't share feelings with wife.	1/16/78	7/20/78
4.	Decreased social and leisure time activities.	1/16/78	5/25/78
5.	Decreased self-esteem.	1/16/78	
6.	Wife depressed.	2/1/78	

INITIAL PLAN

Patient: R.F.J.
1/16/78

Problem # 1: *Feels depressed*

Description (D): Patient says that he has felt "depressed" for the past two months. During this time he has noted decreased appetite, has had difficulty falling asleep, and has taken Dalmane, 30 mgm. at night for sleep, as prescribed by Dr. Smith one month ago. He has noted no weight loss, no decreased libido, and no feelings of hopelessness. He denies suicidal thoughts. No previous history of depression. There is no family history of depressive disorders.

Assessment (A): Patient appears to be suffering from a depression of the reactive type (depressive neurosis). The lack of family history of depression and the relative lack of any biological concomitants of depression weigh against a severe or endogenous depression. I see no evidence of hopelessness or suicidal thoughts.

I believe that this depression is related to problems 2, 3, and 5. It appears that the recent promotion of a younger man has affected his self-esteem, and caused him to devalue himself as a man in relationship to his job and to his marriage.

Plan (P): Goal of treatment will be to decrease his depression and this will be accomplished by treating the patient in psychotherapy aimed at problems 2, 3, and 5. He will initially be seen twice a week.

Problem # 2: *Dissatisfied with job performance*

D: Patient reports that he was passed over for promotion by a younger man two months ago. He felt that this man was "too aggressive." Since that time, he has felt that he has performed less adequately on the job, although he has received no such notice from his supervisor. The patient notes that lately he has been working 50 hours per week as opposed to his previous 60 hours per week. He says he just "doesn't feel like" working longer hours.

A: Patient seems to have some unrealistic expectations of himself and his job. It is questionable whether his long working hours are necessary for adequate job performance. It is possible that his feelings toward his job are colored by comparing himself to his father, who worked two jobs to support the family. There is evidence that the patient feels obligated toward his father to work as hard as he did, and seeks approval from his boss for so doing. Therefore, this problem is also affected by problem # 5, and affects problem # 1.

P: The goal for this problem will be to increase his satisfaction with his job. This will be accomplished by individual psychotherapy. His feeling toward the job in relationship to his father, as well as the reality of his long work hours will be explored. His feelings of anger and frustration toward being passed over for promotion must be explored in terms of the effect on his own lowered self-esteem.

Problem # 3: *Doesn't share feelings with his wife*

D: Patient noted that his wife left the state about two months ago to take care of her sick mother. She has been preoccupied with her mother's illness, and the patient states "I know I should be more supportive of her, but I can't." The patient thinks that things are not right between him and his wife, that he cannot confide in her, that he cannot show his feelings for her (either angry feelings or positive feelings). There has been no change in their sexual relationship, which is apparently satisfactory to them both. The couple have no children because of his wife's fertility problems, according to the patient.

A: This problem seems to be affected by his feelings of depression and lowered self-esteem secondary to his job situation. The decreased social interaction and leisure time activities have also decreased his opportunity for a closer relationship with his wife. It is obvious that he has some underlying anger toward his wife and feels "abandoned" during his job crisis. The wife's concern over her mother may be causing a grief reaction in her that also affects their relationship.

P: To increase his satisfactions in his marriage and his ability to share his feelings with his wife. This will be accomplished through psychotherapy by having him express these feelings of frustration, his feelings of isolation, and increase his ability to confide both positive and angry feelings to his wife. If this is accomplished, it is expected that his wife will be able to support an increase in his self-esteem. A joint session, or session with the wife alone, may be necessary to evaluate the depth of her own grief or depression.

Problem # 4: *Decreased social and leisure time*

D: Patient has noted a decrease in his social and leisure time activities. Prior to the past two months, he enjoyed bowling, but now "doesn't feel like it." He now spends his time watching T.V. He doesn't want his wife to invite friends for dinner because "he doesn't feel like it."

A: This problem is secondary to problem # 1, his feelings of depression, and is also affected by his suppressed anger toward his wife for his feelings of abandonment.

P: Goal is to increase his social interaction and leisure time activities. See plans for problems # 1, 3, and 5.

Problem # 5: *Decreased self-esteem*

D: The patient compared himself unfavorably to his father, and feels that his father liked his brother better than he.

A: This is probably a long-standing problem, but has been increased by the occurrence of the promotion two months ago, and by his wife's concern about her mother. This decrease in self-esteem has directly affected his depression, his attitude toward his job, and his relationship with his wife.

P: Increase his self-esteem in relationship to his job and his marriage. Since this problem is interconnected with problems # 2 and # 1, the plan for this problem will be the same as for those. Whether the longer-standing self-esteem problem can be treated will be evaluated later. The patient will be seen initially twice a week for psychotherapy and a re-evaluation will be done in two months.

Signed:_____

John Frazer, M.D.

PROGRESS NOTE 3/24/78
(TWO MONTH SUMMARY)

Patient: R.F.J.

Problem # 1: *Feels depressed*
    D: Has felt less depressed over past three weeks. Appetite has improved. Still takes Dalmane about twice a week because of sleep difficulty.
    A: Some improvement in depression secondary to progress on problems # 2 and # 5.
    P: Continue twice a week psychotherapy aimed at problems # 2 and # 5.

Problem # 2: *Dissatisfied with job performance*
    D: Has been able to express anger and frustration toward missed promotion. Has connected his dissatisfaction with problem # 5, and feels that some of his problems here are unrealistically connected with past feelings toward father and brother.
    A: Less dissatisfaction with job. Not so certain the promotion was one he really wanted.
    P: Continue plan as before, concentrating on problem # 5, and its relationship to this problem

Problem # 3: *Doesn't share feelings with wife*
    D: Met wife with patient's permission on 2/1/78. She has been involved with her own concern about her mother's terminal illness. She feels she has not been very supportive of husband and vice-versa. Patient has slowly been able to recognize her grief and concern, and is less angry at her perceived abandonment of him. (See problem # 6.)
    A: Still a problem, but progress being made in this area.
    P: No further sessions with wife anticipated at this point. Emphasize work on problem # 5 in psychotherapy.

Problem # 4:   *Decreased social and leisure time*
      D: Patient and wife still do very little together outside the home. He has gone bowling only once in the past three months. They have gone out to dinner together twice.
      A: Slight progress. Considering the crises both are experiencing, their level of social contact may be appropriate.
      P: No current direct plan for this problem

Problem # 5:   *Decreased self-esteem*
      D: See problems # 1, # 2, and # 3.
      A: Some progress. This problem is the central focus in psychotherapy at present, since it directly affects problems # 1, # 2, # 3, and # 4.
      P: Continue twice a week psychotherapy and re-evaluate in two months to see if further work is necessary.

Problem # 6:   *Wife depressed*
      D: See (D) under problem # 3. She shows difficulty concentrating and loss of interest except in her mother's condition.
      A: This is a problem for patient because of his need for her support.
      P: Will help him recognize her depression as her problem, and that it does not mean she thinks less of him. As he improves, he can be more supportive of her problems.

Signed: _____

John Frazer, M.D.

TERMINATION NOTE 8/5/78

Patient is a 46-year-old married man, referred by Dr. Jonas Smith on 1/16/78, because of depression of two months duration.

The following problems were identified and treated:
1. *Feels depressed*
   Patient had felt depressed for two months, with decreased appetite and some insomnia. This was felt to be a depressive neurosis secondary to problems # 2, # 3, and # 5. Responded well to twice a week psychotherapy for four months and once a week psychotherapy for five weeks, totalling 35 sessions. Patient will call in three months to give me a progress report.

2. *Dissatisfied with job performance*
   This problem preceded problem # 1, and coincided with the patient's being passed over for promotion. This problem was felt to affect problem # 5, and was related to patient's feelings about his father and brother. He is currently working 45 hours a week, and feels much more satisfied with his job.

3. *Doesn't share feelings with his wife*
   This problem occurred when wife became very involved with her terminally

ill mother at the same time problem # 2 was occurring. Was felt to affect problems # 1, # 4, and # 5. Session with wife on 2/1/78 revealed her own grief about her mother. As patient became less depressed and more satisfied with his job, his self-esteem improved and he is better able to support his wife and share his own feelings with her.

4. *Decreased social and leisure time*
Patient had decreased personal leisure time activities as well as social time with wife secondary to problems # 1, # 3, and # 5. As these problems improved, the patient's activities increased, and both he and his wife are more socially active.

5. *Decreased self-esteem*
This problem stemmed from his past relationship with his brother and father, and was increased by problems # 2 and # 3. As these problems improved, patient was able to see that he was expecting more support from his wife and supervisor than he needed, was able to look at his job more realistically, and is now feeling more worthwhile as an employee and as a husband.

6. *Wife depressed*
Interview with wife revealed her depression over her mother's illness. As patient became more able to recognize this, it became less of a problem for him although it is still a problem for her. He is now more supportive of her, however.

Patient will call with a progress report in three months.

Signed:_____

John Frazer, M.D.

8. Conventional Clinical Record: Initial Evaluation and Treatment Plan

Patient:	R.F.J.
Birth date:	3/31/31
Referred by:	Dr. Jonas Smith
	Medical Arts Clinic

1/16/78

Patient is a 46-year-old married man, referred by his physician for evaluation of depression.

Patient states that he has felt "depressed" for the past two months. During this time, he has noted decreased interest in his job and some decreased appetite. He has had difficulty falling asleep and has taken sleeping pills regularly for the past month. He has noted no weight loss, no decreased libido, and no feelings of hopelessness. Denies suicidal thoughts. No previous history of such feelings, or previous contact with a mental health professional.

Onset of these symptoms corresponds to the time he was passed over for promotion for a younger man whom he feels is "too aggressive." In addition, shortly thereafter, his wife went to another state to take care of her sick mother for two weeks. "Things haven't been right between us since." Patient says that his wife has been more concerned about her mother's failing health. "I can understand her concern, and I should be more supportive, but I can't."

Patient denies alcohol or drug abuse. Has 1 to 2 drinks at parties. Has taken only medications prescribed by physician. (Has taken Dalmane, 30 mgm. at night for sleep since prescribed by Dr. Smith one month ago.)

Relevant Past History

Patient raised in this state. Father was a laborer. He "worked hard to put us through school." Died of a heart attack at age 54, immediately after patient, age 22, graduated college (B.A. in business administration). Patient took job with insurance company, where he has worked since, rather than wait for a better job because he felt obligated to support his mother.

183

Father worked two jobs to support family, and patient feels this contributed to his death. "He sacrificed for us." "I'll never be the man he was." Never felt emotionally close to father. Mother died four years ago at age 72, of a stroke. Patient shows sadness and cries when speaking of her death. "She worked hard too, bringing us up. She was the one we could bring our problems to."

Patient's only sibling, a brother, 50 years old, is a vice-president of a chemical manufacturing corporation. "He was always the go-getter of the family. He's not the kind anyone can get close to. He's his own man." Patient and brother have had little contact since the death of their mother.

No family history of depression or other emotional disorders.

Current Functioning

Job: Patient feels he has performed less adequately on the job for past three months. Although he has had no complaints from his boss, he suspects that his boss is dissatisfied with his work. Patient cannot be specific about how he might be performing less adequately, except that he is now spending less time (50 hours vs. 60 hours/week) working.

Marriage: Doesn't feel as close to his wife as before. Doesn't confide in her. Holds back his feelings toward wife, both affectionate and angry during the past few months. No change in sexual relationship over past five years. Both seem satisfied, according to patient. No children. She had fertility problems, according to patient.

Social Relationships - Leisure Time: In the past, patient has enjoyed bowling with friends at work. More recently, "hasn't felt like it. Watch T.V. some." His wife has wanted to invite friends over for dinner, but patient "hasn't felt like it."

Physical Health

According to report from Dr. Smith, patient is in good physical health. No evidence of organic disease to account for symptoms.

Mental Status

Looks his age. Wearing tie and sport jacket. Slumps in chair. Appears anxious. States that he feels depressed. Cries briefly several times during interview, but quickly changes subject. Shows deference to examiner. Thought content in keeping with depressed mood: "Lack of enjoyment," "don't feel like it." Has good memory for dates and times, and therefore no formal evaluation of sensorium or calculation ability was performed. Made no loose associations or bizarre statements. Shows some insight in recognizing that his feelings of depression are related to his job and recent events in his marriage, although he is not clear of the relationship.

Assessment

Patient is experiencing a depressive syndrome, most likely of the reactive type (depressive neurosis). The lack of family history of depression and the relative lack of the biological concomitants of depression (e.g. severe anorexia, diurnal variation in mood, decreased libido, or impotency, etc.) weigh against a severe or endogenous type of depression. I see no evidence of hopelessness or suicidal thoughts which might necessitate hospitalization.

Psychodynamically, it appears that his resentment at being passed over for promotion, his unrecognized anger at his wife for "leaving" him when he needed her support, and his comparing himself unfavorably with his brother have all combined to decrease his self-esteem to the point of self-blame and resulting depression. He feels unrewarded for his hard work, and may be unrealistically dependent on the recognition of others for his own self-esteem.

Plan: Psychotherapy twice a week.

Goals: 1. To provide him the opportunity to express his anger regarding the missed promotion.
2. To allow him to express his frustration at his wife in psychotherapy so that this communication channel can be opened.
3. To help him re-evaluate his own image of himself vis-a-vis his job and his brother.
4. To assess the necessity of his working 60 hours a week and the relative lack of satisfactions in his life.

The necessity for twice-a-week psychotherapy will be re-evaluated in two months.

Signed:_____

John Frazer, M.D.

PROGRESS NOTE 3/24/78
(TWO MONTH SUMMARY)

Patient: R.F.J.

Patient has been seen twice weekly for psychotherapy. He has established good rapport with therapist and has made progress toward some of the goals previously established.

His anger and frustration concerning his job have been expressed vocally and with tears. He has connected his concern over the missed promotion with his feeling that his father thought that his brother was more capable than he. In expressing these concerns, the patient has questioned whether he actually wanted the promotion itself, or only as proof of his boss' regard. He now feels less concerned about his job performance.

He has been less able to recognize his feelings of being abandoned by his wife during a time when he wanted her support. Inquiry into this area has resulted in defensiveness and sarcasm. I plan to go slowly in this area. It is obvious that the support of his wife is important to him and he has difficulty recognizing his ambivalent feelings toward her.

It appears that his work is an attempt to expiate some of his guilt over his father's sacrifice for his children and his anger toward his father for seemingly preferring his brother to him. It is doubtful that these conflicts can be resolved in a relatively short amount of time, but this resolution may not be necessary to deal with his depression.

Conclusions

Patient seems somewhat less depressed, although the symptoms are still affecting his marriage and his job.

Plan: Concentrate on helping him deal with his feelings toward his wife, and explore possibility of progress in dealing with his unresolved guilt about his father's death. Continue psychotherapy twice a week. Review again in two months.

Signed: _____

John Frazer, M.D.

Appendixes

Patient: R.F.J.

Patient was referred on 1/16/78 by his family physician, Dr. Jonas Smith, because of depression of two months duration. His symptoms were affecting his work and his marriage. Patient's symptoms were related to recent events at work and the illness of a relative, as well as with some difficulty in expressing his feelings of frustration about these situations.

He was treated twice a week for the first four months and once a week for the last five weeks, for a total of 35 sessions. Treatment consisted of individual psychotherapy aimed at helping him better cope with his frustrations and somewhat unrealistic expectations of himself. He improved in his ability to deal with job requirements, began to enjoy his job and his marriage more, and found satisfaction in more leisure time activities. He now works 45 hours per week, and spends his weekends with his wife in mutually satisfying activities.

With this improvement, the patient's depression is no longer a problem. He will call me again in three months to give a progress report. Otherwise, he is discharged.

Signed:_____

John Frazer, M.D.

9. Mental Health Practitioner Specialties

Credit: Derived from APA Directory Survey, 1978, and reproduced by permission of American Psychological Association, 1200 Seventeenth Street N.W., Washington, D.C. 20036.

DEVELOPMENTAL (Life-span)

Infancy
Childhood
    Perception
    Learning
    Concepts & Language
    Abilities
    Emotional Development
    Motivational Development
    Personality
    Social Behavior
    Parent-Child & Family Relations
    Child Abuse
    Physical/Motor Development
    Children's Literature and Art
    Basic Reading Processes
Adolescence
Adulthood
Aging
Developmental Theory
  & Methodology
Development of the Mentally
  Retarded
Development of the Physically
  Handicapped
    Development of the Blind
    Development of the Deaf

Thanatology
Cognition

PERSONALITY

Personality Traits & Processes
    Behavior Correlates
    Culture & Personality
Creativity
Intelligence & Measurement of
  Intelligence
Individual Differences
Personality Measurement
    Inventories & Rating Scales
    Projective Techniques
    Rorschach Tests
Personality Assessment
Social Learning & Personality
    Self Concept & Role Concept
    Learning

SOCIAL

Interpersonal Processes
    Influence & Communication
    Interpersonal Relations
    Social Perception & Motivation
    Aggression

Appendixes

Intra & Inter Group Processes
    Group Conflict & Attitudes
    Influence & Communication
    Group Decision Making &
      Performance
    Group Structure
    Leadership
    T-Groups/Sensitivity/Encounter
Communication
    Mass Media Communication
    Language
    Nonverbal & Paraverbal
      Communication
Attitudes & Opinions
    Formation & Change
    Influence & Behavior
    Survey & Measurement
    Attribution Theory
Values & Moral Behavior
Alcohol Use
Drug Use
Smoking
Sexual Behavior
    Birth Control
    Sexual Life Styles
    Sex Roles/Differences
Human Ecology
Psychology & the Arts
Culture & Social Processes
    Ethnology
    Socioeconomic Structure &
      Roles
    Religion
    Cross Cultural Comparison
    Family
    Social Change & Programs
    Crime Reduction
Psychology of Ethnic Groups

CLINICAL

Psychotherapy
    Client-Therapist Interaction
    Behavior & Conditioning
      Therapy
    Group Therapy
    Drug Therapy
    Hypnotherapy
    Special & Adjunctive Therapy
    Adolescent Therapy
    Gestalt Therapy
    Individual & Group Therapy
    Behavior Modification
    Primal Therapy

Adlerian Therapy
Applied Behavior Analysis
Bioenergetic Therapy
Biofeedback
Existential Therapy
Feminist Therapy
Jungian Therapy
Psychodrama
Rational-Emotive Therapy
Reichian Therapy
Sex/Marital Therapy
Transactional Therapy
Transpersonal Psychology
Hypnosis/Hypnotherapy
Clinical Child Psychology
    Childhood Disorders
    Assessment
    Family Therapy
    Art/Play Therapy
    Institutions & Programs
    Child Therapy
    Autism
    Learning Disabilities
    Parent Education
Psychoanalysis
    Psychoanalytic Theory
Psychodiagnosis
Psychopathology
Behavior & Mental Disorders
    Alcoholism
    Crime
    Drug Abuse
    Sexual Inadequacy &
      Dysfunction
    Juvenile Delinquency
    Neurosis & Emotional Disorder
    Psychosis
    Schizophrenia
    Suicide
    Psychopathic & Character
      Disorders
    Obesity/Aphagia
Neurological Disorder
    Brain Damage
    Epilepsy
    Clinical Neuropsychology
Mentally Retarded
    Learning & Motor Ability
    Training & Vocational
      Rehabilitation
Speech Disorder
Psychosomatic Disorder
Medical Psychology
Gerontology

Clinical Community Services
Hospital Care & Institutionalization
Applied Clinical Research
Reading Disorders
Physically Handicapped
    Disabled
    Blind
    Deaf
Death & Dying
Program Evaluation

COMMUNITY

Community Mental Health
    Family Therapy
    Crisis Intervention & Therapy
    Day Hospital Practices
    Small Group Processes
    Mental Health Services
    Community Mental Health
        Consultation
    Community Mental Health
        Services Planning
    Community Mental Health
        Administration
Community Development
    Community Leadership
    Manpower Training (non-
        professional)
    Community Organization
    Social Policy Analysis
    Social Program Planning
    Community Advocacy
Research & Training
Counselor Education
Rehabilitation Administration

COUNSELING
(see also School & Industrial)

General Counseling
    Rehabilitation Counseling
    Vocational Counseling
    Educational Counseling
    Employee Counseling
    Marriage & Family Counseling
    Personal or Adjustment
        Counseling
    Pastoral Counseling
    Counseling, Disabled,
        Handicapped
    Counseling, Employment
Counseling Methods & Processes
    Individual & Group Counseling

Testing
Diagnosis & Assessment
Psychotherapy
Test Validation & Counseling Effec-
    tiveness
Counseling Theory
Counseling Education

SCHOOL
(see also Counseling)

School Counseling
    Behavior Problems
    Emotional Adjustment
    Learning Difficulties
    Physically Handicapped
    Gifted Children
    Preschool Children
Methods & Processes
    Testing
    Diagnosis & Assessment
    Therapeutic Processes
    Student-Teacher Relationship
    Parent-child Relationship
Child Growth & Development
Administration of Psychological Ser-
    vices
School Organization & Administration
Psychoeducational Diagnosis

EDUCATIONAL

School Learning, Theory &
    Processes
Teacher Selection & Training
Teaching Methods
    Teaching Machines
    Programmed Instruction
    Teaching Aids
Special Education
    Disadvantaged
    Gifted
    Emotionally Disturbed
    Mentally Deficient
    Physically Handicapped
Preschool Education & Day Care
Curriculum Development/Evaluation
Special Programs (Compensatory,
    Remedial)
Educational Measurement & Evalua-
    tion
    Intelligence
    Aptitude & Adjustment

Readiness
School Learning Achievement
Educational Research
Educational Technology
College/University Teaching
Continuing/Adult Education

ENGINEERING

Work Performance/Schedules
Stress Factors (Fatigue, Monotony)
Work Performance Improvement (Time & Motion Study)
Accident Prevention, Safety
Work Environments
Noise & Vibration
Special Environments (Space, Underwater)
Man-Machine Systems (Analysis & Design)
Human Factors
Displays & Controls

Equipment Design
Instructional Materials & Training

INDUSTRIAL & ORGANIZATIONAL
(see also Counseling)

Personnel
Selection & Placement
Career Development & Training
Performance Evaluation
Job Satisfaction, Morale & Attitudes
Retirement
Management & Organization
Organizational Behavior
Labor-Management Relations
Position & Task Analysis
Compensation
Human Relations
Organization Development
Employee/Vocational Counseling
Environment & Quality of Life

Ethical Standards
of Psychologists

(1977 Revision)

American Psychological Association

Appendixes

Published by the American Psychological Association, 1200 Seventeenth Street, N.W., Washington, D.C. 20036. Copyright © 1977 American Psychological Association, Inc.

Ethical Standards of Psychologists [1]

Climaxing nine years of work by several task forces and the Committee on Scientific and Professional Ethics and Conduct (CSPEC), draft #11 of the Ethical Standards of Psychologists went to the Council of Representatives at its January 28-30, 1977 meeting. A number of changes were made in the document by Council, resulting in draft #12, which was adopted on January 30th as printed below.

Because the Council could not agree on several sections of Principle 5 (Confidentiality), the final action was to approve the final revised draft with the exception of this principle. The old principle (formerly Principle 6 in the Ethical Standards as printed in the 1975 *Biographical Directory*) will hold until a revision has been adopted by Council.

Council comments and suggestions applicable to this section are now being solicited by CSPEC. Council also directed the Committee to take into account the forthcoming report of the Task Force on Privacy and Confidentiality, as well as upcoming federal regulations covering similar matters. APA members having specific wording changes to suggest may send them to Brenda Gurel, Secretary, CSPEC, APA, 1200 Seventeenth Street, N.W., Washington, D.C. 20036.

PREAMBLE

Psychologists[1,2] *respect the dignity and worth of the individual and honor the preservation and protection of fundamental human rights. They are committed to increasing knowledge of human behavior and of people's understanding of themselves and others and to the utilization of such knowledge for the promotion of human welfare. While pursuing these endeavors, they make every effort to protect the welfare of those who seek their services or of any human being or animal that may be the object of study. They use their skills only for purposes consistent with these values and do not knowingly permit their misuse by others. While demanding for themselves freedom of inquiry and communication, psychologists accept the responsibility this freedom requires: competence,*

objectivity in the application of skills and concern for the best interests of clients, colleagues, and society in general. In the pursuit of these ideals, psychologists subscribe to principles in the following areas: 1. Responsibility, 2. Competence, 3. Moral and Legal Standards, 4. Public Statements, 5. Confidentiality, 6. Welfare of the Consumer, 7. Professional Relationships, 8. Utilization of Assessment Techniques, and 9. Pursuit of Research Activities.

PRINCIPLE 1. RESPONSIBILITY

In their commitment to the understanding of human behavior, psychologists value objectivity and integrity, and in providing services they maintain the highest standards of their profession. They accept responsibility for the consequences of their work and make every effort to insure that their services are used appropriately.

a. As scientists, psychologists accept the ultimate responsibility for selecting appropriate areas and methods most relevant to these areas. They plan their research in ways to minimize the possibility that their findings will be misleading. They provide thorough discussion of the limitations of their data and alternative hypotheses, especially where their work touches on social policy or might be construed to the detriment of persons in specific age, sex, ethnic, socioeconomic or other social groups. In publishing reports of their work, they never suppress disconfirming data. Psychologists take credit only for the work they have actually done.

Psychologists clarify in advance with all appropriate persons or agencies the expectations for sharing and utilizing research data. They avoid dual relationships which may limit objectivity, whether political or monetary, so that interference with data, human participants, and milieu is kept to a minimum.

b. As employees of an institution or agency, psychologists have the responsibility of remaining alert to and attempting to moderate institutional pressures that may distort reports of psychological findings or impede their proper use.

c. As members of governmental or other organizational bodies, psychologists remain accountable as individuals to the highest standards of their profession.

[1] Approved by the Council of Representatives, January 30, 1977. Reprinted from the APA "Monitor," March 1977.

[2] A student of psychology who assumes the role of a psychologist shall be considered a psychologist for the purpose of this code of ethics.

d. As teachers, psychologists recognize their primary obligation to help others acquire knowledge and skill. They maintain high standards of scholarship and objectivity by presenting psychological information fully and accurately.

e. As practitioners, psychologists know that they bear a heavy social responsibility because their recommendations and professional actions may alter the lives of others. They are alert to personal, social, organizational, financial, or political situations or pressures that might lead to misuse of their influence.

f. Psychologists provide adequate and timely evaluations to employees, trainees, students, and others whose work they supervise.

PRINCIPLE 2.
COMPETENCE

The maintenance of high standards of professional competence is a responsibility shared by all psychologists in the interest of the public and the profession as a whole. Psychologists recognize the boundaries of their competence and the limitations of their techniques and only provide services, use techniques, or offer opinions as professionals that meet recognized standards. Psychologists maintain knowledge of current scientific and professional information related to the services they render.

a. Psychologists accurately represent their competence, education, training and experience. Psychologists claim as evidence of professional qualifications only those degrees obtained from institutions acceptable under the Bylaws and Rules of Council of the American Psychological Association.

b. As teachers, psychologists perform their duties on the basis of careful preparation so that their instruction is accurate, current and scholarly.

c. Psychologists recognize the need for continuing education and are open to new procedures and changes in expectations and values over time. They recognize differences among people, such as those that may be associated with age, sex, socioeconomic, and ethnic backgrounds. Where relevant, they obtain training, experience, or counsel to assure competent service or research relating to such persons.

d. Psychologists with the responsibility for decisions involving individuals or policies based on test results have an understanding of psychological or educational measurement, validation problems and other test research.

e. Psychologists recognize that their effectiveness depends in part upon their ability to maintain effective interpersonal relations, and that aberrations on their part may interfere with their abilities. They refrain from undertaking any activity in which their personal problems are likely to lead to inadequate professional services or harm to a client; or, if engaged in such activity when they become aware of their personal problems, they seek competent professional assistance to determine whether they should suspend, terminate or limit the scope of their professional and/or scientific activities.

PRINCIPLE 3.
MORAL AND LEGAL STANDARDS

Psychologists' moral, ethical and legal standards of behavior are a personal matter to the same degree as they are for any other citizen, except as these may compromise the fulfillment of their professional responsibilities, or reduce the trust in psychology or psychologists held by the general public. Regarding their own behavior, psychologists should be aware of the prevailing community standards and of the possible impact upon the quality of professional services provided by their conformity to or deviation from these standards. Psychologists are also aware of the possible impact of their public behavior upon the ability of colleagues to perform their professional duties.

a. Psychologists as teachers are aware of the diverse backgrounds of students and, when dealing with topics that may give offense, treat the material objectively and present it in a manner for which the student is prepared.

b. As employees, psychologists refuse to participate in practices inconsistent with legal, moral and ethical standards regarding the treatment of employees or of the public. For example, psychologists will not condone practices that are inhumane or that result in illegal or otherwise unjustifiable discrimination on the basis of race, age, sex, religion, or national origin in hiring, promotion, or training.

c. In providing psychological services,

psychologists avoid any action that will violate or diminish the legal and civil rights of clients or of others who may be affected by their actions.

As practitioners, psychologists remain abreast of relevant federal, state, local, and agency regulations and Association standards of practice concerning the conduct of their practice. They are concerned with developing such legal and quasi-legal regulations as best serve the public interest and in changing such existing regulations as are not beneficial to the interests of the public and the profession.

d. As researchers, psychologists remain abreast of relevant federal and state regulations concerning the conduct of research with human participants or animals.

PRINCIPLE 4.
PUBLIC STATEMENTS

Public statements, announcements of services, and promotional activities of psychologists serve the purpose of providing sufficient information to aid the consumer public in making informed judgments and choices. Psychologists represent accurately and objectively their professional qualifications, affiliations, and functions, as well as those of the institutions or organizations with which they or the statements may be associated. In public statements providing psychological information or professional opinions or providing information about the availability of psychological products and services, psychologists take full account of the limits and uncertainties of present psychological knowledge and techniques.

a. When announcing professional services, psychologists limit the information to: name, highest relevant academic degree conferred, date and type of certification or licensure, diplomate status, address, telephone number, office hours, and a brief listing of the type of psychological services offered. Such statements are descriptive of services provided but not evaluative as to their quality or uniqueness. They do not contain testimonials by quotation or by implication. They do not claim uniqueness of skills or methods unless determined by acceptable and public scientific evidence.

b. In announcing the availability of psychological services or products, psychologists do not display any affiliations with an orga-

nization in a manner that falsely implies the sponsorship or certification of that organization. In particular and for example, psychologists do not offer APA membership or fellowship as evidence of qualification. They do not name their employer or professional associations unless the services are in fact to be provided by or under the responsible, direct supervision and continuing control of such organizations or agencies.

c. Announcements of "personal growth groups" give a clear statement of purpose and the nature of the experiences to be provided. The education, training and experience of the psychologists are appropriately specified.

d. Psychologists associated with the development or promotion of psychological devices, books, or other products offered for commercial sale make every effort to insure that announcements and advertisements are presented in a professional, scientifically acceptable, and factually informative manner.

e. Psychologists do not participate for personal gain in commercial announcements recommending to the general public the purchase or use or any proprietary or single-source product or service.

f. Psychologists who interpret the science of psychology or the services of psychologists to the general public accept the obligation to present the material fairly and accurately, avoiding misrepresentation through sensationalism, exaggeration or superficiality. Psychologists are guided by the primary obligation to aid the public in forming their own informed judgments, opinions and choices.

g. As teachers, psychologists insure that statements in catalogs and course outlines are accurate and sufficient, particularly in terms of subject matter to be covered, bases for evaluating progress, and nature of course experiences. Announcements or brochures describing workshops, seminars, or other educational programs accurately represent intended audience and eligibility requirements, educational objectives, and nature of the material to be covered, as well as the education, training and experience of the psychologists presenting the programs, and any fees involved. Public announcements soliciting subjects for research, and in which clinical services or other professional services are offered as an inducement, make clear the nature of the services as well as the costs and other obligations to be accepted by the human participants of the research.

h. Psychologists accept the obligation to correct others who may represent the psychologist's professional qualifications or associations with products or services in a manner incompatible with these guidelines.

i. Psychological services for the purpose of diagnosis, treatment or personal advice are provided only in the context of a professional relationship, and are not given by means of public lectures or demonstrations, newspaper or magazine articles, radio or television programs, mail, or similar media.

PRINCIPLE 5.
CONFIDENTIALITY

Safeguarding information about an individual that has been obtained by the psychologist in the course of his teaching, practice, or investigation is a primary obligation of the psychologist. Such information is not communicated to others unless certain important conditions are not met.

a. Information received in confidence is revealed only after most careful deliberation and when there is clear and imminent danger to an individual or to society, and then only to appropriate professional workers or public authorities.

b. Information obtained in clinical or consulting relationships, or evaluative data concerning children, students, employees, and others are discussed only for professional purposes and only with persons clearly concerned with the case. Written and oral reports should present only data germane to the purposes of the evaluation and every effort should be made to avoid undue invasion of privacy.

c. Clinical and other materials are used in classroom teaching and writing only when the identity of the persons involved is adequately disguised.

d. The confidentiality of professional communications about individuals is maintained. Only when the originator and other persons involved give their express permission is a confidential professional communication shown to the individual concerned. The psychologist is responsible for informing the client of the limits of the confidentiality.

e. Only after explicit permission has been granted is the identity of research subjects published. When data have been published without permission for identification, the psy-

chologist assumes responsibility for adequately disguising their sources.

f. The psychologist makes provisions for the maintenance of confidentiality in the prevention and ultimate disposition of confidential records.

PRINCIPLE 6.
WELFARE OF THE CONSUMER

Psychologists respect the integrity and protect the welfare of the people and groups with whom they work. When there is a conflict of interest between the client and the psychologist's employing institution, psychologists clarify the nature and direction of their loyalties and responsibilities and keep all parties informed of their commitments. Psychologists fully inform consumers as to the purpose and nature of an evaluative, treatment, educational or training procedure, and they freely acknowledge that clients, students, or participants in research have freedom of choice with regard to participation.

a. Psychologists are continually cognizant of their own needs and of their inherently powerful position *vis a vis* clients, in order to avoid exploiting their trust and dependency. Psychologists make every effort to avoid dual relationships with clients and/or relationships which might impair their professional judgment or increase the risk of client exploitation. Examples of such dual relationships include treating employees, supervisees, close friends or relatives. Sexual intimacies with clients are unethical.

b. Where demands of an organization on psychologists go beyond reasonable conditions of employment, psychologists recognize possible conflicts of interest that may arise. When such conflicts occur, psychologists clarify the nature of the conflict and inform all parties of the nature and direction of the loyalties and responsibilities involved.

c. When acting as a supervisor, trainer, researcher, or employer, psychologists accord informed choice, confidentiality, due process, and protection from physical and mental harm to their subordinates in such relationships.

d. Financial arrangements in professional practice are in accord with professional standards that safeguard the best interests of the client and that are clearly understood by the client in advance of billing. Psychologists are responsible for assisting clients in finding needed services in those instances where payment of the usual fee would be a hardship. No commission, rebate, or other form of remuneration may be given or received for referral of clients for professional services, whether by an individual or by an agency. Psychologists willingly contribute a portion of their services to work for which they receive little or no financial return.

e. The psychologist attempts to terminate a clinical or consulting relationship when it is reasonably clear that the consumer is not benefiting from it. Psychologists who find that their services are being used by employers in a way that is not beneficial to the participants or to employees who may be affected, or to significant others, have the responsibility to make their observations known to the responsible persons and to propose modification or termination of the engagement.

PRINCIPLE 7. PROFESSIONAL RELATIONSHIPS

Psychologists act with due regard for the needs, special competencies and obligations of their colleagues in psychology and other professions. Psychologists respect the prerogatives and obligations of the institutions or organizations with which they are associated.

a. Psychologists understand the areas of competence of related professions, and make full use of all the professional, technical, and administrative resources that best serve the interests of consumers. The absence of formal relationships with other professional workers does not relieve psychologists from the responsibility of securing for their clients the best possible professional service nor does it relieve them from the exercise of foresight, diligence, and tact in obtaining the complementary or alternative assistance needed by clients.

b. Psychologists know and take into account the traditions and practices of other professional groups with which they work and cooperate fully with members of such groups. If a consumer is receiving services from another professional, psychologists do not offer their services directly to the consumer without first informing the professional person already involved so that the risk of confusion and conflict for the consumer can be avoided.

c. Psychologists who employ or supervise other professionals or professionals in training accept the obligation to facilitate their further professional development by providing suitable working conditions, consultation, and experience opportunities.

d. As employees of organizations providing psychological services, or as independent psychologists serving clients in an organizational context, psychologists seek to support the integrity, reputation and proprietary rights of the host organization. When it is judged necessary in a client's interest to question the organization's programs or policies, psychologists attempt to effect change by constructive action within the organization before disclosing confidential information acquired in their professional roles.

e. In the pursuit of research, psychologists give sponsoring agencies, host institutions, and publication channels the same respect and opportunity for giving informed consent that they accord to individual research participants. They are aware of their obligation to future research workers and insure that host institutions are given adequate information about the research and proper acknowledgement of their contributions.

f. Publication credit is assigned to all those who have contributed to a publication in proportion to their contribution. Major contributions of a professional character made by several persons to a common project are recognized by joint authorship, with the experimenter or author who made the principal contribution identified and listed first. Minor contributions of a professional character, extensive clerical or similar nonprofessional assistance, and other minor contributions are acknowledged in footnotes or in an introductory statement. Acknowledgement through specific citations is made for unpublished as well as published material that has directly influenced the research or writing. A psychologist who compiles and edits material of others for publication publishes the material in the name of the originating group, if any, and with his/her own name appearing as chairperson or editor. All contributors are to be acknowledged and named.

g. When a psychologist violates ethical standards, psychologists who know first-hand of such activities should, if possible, attempt to rectify the situation. Failing an informal solution, psychologists bring such unethical activities to the attention of the appropriate local, state, and/or national committee on professional ethics, standards, and practices.

h. Members of the Association cooperate with duly constituted committees of the Association, in particular and for example, the Committee on Scientific and Professional Ethics and Conduct, and the Committee on Professional Standards Review, by responding to inquiries promptly and completely. Members taking longer than 30 days to respond to such inquiries shall have the burden of demonstrating that they acted with "reasonable promptness." Members also have a similar responsibility to respond with reasonable promptness to inquiries from duly constituted state association ethics committees and professional standards review committees.

PRINCIPLE 8. UTILIZATION OF ASSESSMENT TECHNIQUES

In the development, publication, and utilization of psychological assessment techniques, psychologists observe relevant APA standards. Persons examined have the right to know the results, the interpretations made, and, where appropriate, the original data on which final judgments were based. Test users avoid imparting unnecessary information which would compromise test security, but they provide requested information that explains the basis for decisions that may adversely affect that person or that person's dependents.

a. The client has the right to have and the psychologist has the responsibility to provide explanations of the nature and the purposes of the test and the test results in language that the client can understand, unless, as in some employment or school settings, there is an explicit exception to this right agreed upon in advance. When the explanations are to be provided by others, the psychologist establishes procedures for providing adequate explanations.

b. When a test is published or otherwise made available for operational use, it is accompanied by a manual (or other published or readily available information) that fully describes the development of the test, the rationale, and evidence of validity and reliability. The test manual explicitly states the purposes and applications for which the test is recommended and identifies special qualifications required to administer the test and to interpret it properly. Test manuals provide complete information regarding the characteristics of the normative population.

c. In reporting test results, psychologists indicate any reservations regarding validity or reliability resulting from testing circumstances or inappropriateness of the test norms for the person tested. Psychologists strive to insure that the test results and their interpretations are not misused by others.

d. Psychologists accept responsibility for removing from clients' files test score information that has become obsolete, lest such information be misused or misconstrued to the disadvantage of the person tested.

e. Psychologists offering test scoring and interpretation services are able to demonstrate that the validity of the programs and procedures used in arriving at interpretations are based on appropriate evidence. The public offering of an automated test interpretation service is considered as a professional-to-professional consultation. The psychologist makes every effort to avoid misuse of test reports.

PRINCIPLE 9. PURSUIT OF RESEARCH ACTIVITIES

The decision to undertake research should rest upon a considered judgment by the individual psychologist about how best to contribute to psychological science and to human welfare. Psychologists carry out their investigations with respect for the people who participate and with concern for their dignity and welfare.

a. In planning a study the investigator has the responsibility to make a careful evaluation of its ethical acceptability, taking into account the following additional principles for research with human beings. To the extent that this appraisal, weighing scientific and humane values, suggests a compromise of any principle, the investigator incurs an increasingly serious obligation to seek ethical advice and to observe stringent safeguards to protect the rights of the human research participants.

b. Responsibility for the establishment and maintenance of acceptable ethical practice in research always remains with the individual investigator. The investigator is also responsible for the ethical treatment of research participants by collaborators, assistants, students, and employees, all of whom, however, incur parallel obligations.

c. Ethical practice requires the investigator to inform the participant of all features of the research that might reasonably be expected to influence willingness to participate, and to explain all other aspects of the research about which the participant inquires. Failure to make full disclosure imposes additional force to the investigator's abiding responsibility to protect the welfare and dignity of the research participant.

d. Openness and honesty are essential characteristics of the relationship between investigator and research participant. When the methodological requirements of a study necessitate concealment or deception, the investigator is required to insure as soon as possible the participant's understanding of the reasons for this action and of a sufficient justification for the procedures employed.

e. Ethical practice requires the investigator to respect the individual's freedom to decline to participate in or withdraw from research. The obligation to protect this freedom requires special vigilance when the investigator is in a position of power over the participant, as, for example, when the participant is a student, client, employee, or otherwise is in a dual relationship with the investigator.

f. Ethically acceptable research begins with the establishment of a clear and fair agreement between the investigator and the research participant that clarifies the responsibilities of each. The investigator has the obligation to honor all promises and commitments included in that agreement.

g. The ethical investigator protects participants from physical and mental discomfort, harm, and danger. If a risk of such consequences exists, the investigator is required to inform the participant of that fact, secure consent before proceeding, and take all possible measures to minimize distress. A research procedure must not be used if it is likely to cause serious or lasting harm to a participant.

h. After the data are collected, the investigator provides the participant with information about the nature of the study and to remove any misconceptions that may have arisen. Where scientific or human values justify delaying or withholding information, the investigator acquires a special responsibility to assure that there are no damaging consequences for the participant.

i. When research procedures may result in undesirable consequences for the individual participant, the investigator has the responsibility to detect and remove or correct these consequences, including, where relevant, long-term after effects.

j. Information obtained about the individual research participants during the course of an investigation is confidential unless otherwise agreed in advance. When the possibility exists that others may obtain access to such information, this possibility, together with the plans for protecting confidentiality, be explained to the participants as part of the procedure for obtaining informed consent.

k. A psychologist using animals in research adheres to the provisions of the Rules Regarding Animals, drawn up by the Committee on Precautions and Standards in Animal Experimentation and adopted by the American Psychological Association.

l. Investigations of human participants using drugs should be conducted only in such settings as clinics, hospitals, or research facilities maintaining appropriate safeguards for the participants.

REFERENCES

Psychologists are responsible for knowing about and acting in accord with the standards and positions of the APA, as represented in such official documents as the following:

American Association of University Professors. Statement on Principles on Academic Freedom and Tenure. *Policy Documents & Report*, 1977, 1-4.

American Psychological Association. *Guidelines for Psychologists for the Use of Drugs in Research.* Washington, D.C.: Author, 1971.

American Psychological Association. *Principles for the Care and Use of Animals.* Washington, D.C.: Author, 1971.

American Psychological Association. Guidelines for conditions of employment of psychologists. *American Psychologist*, 1972, *27*, 331-334.

American Psychological Association. Guidelines for psychologists conducting growth groups. *American Psychologist*, 1973, *28*, 933.

American Psychological Association. *Ethical Principles in the Conduct of Research with Human Participants.* Washington, D.C.: Author, 1973.

American Psychological Association. *Standards for Educational and Psychological Tests.* Washington, D.C.: Author, 1974.

American Psychological Association. *Standards for Providers of Psychological Services.* Washington, D.C.: Author, 1977.

Committee on Scientific and Professional Ethics and Conduct. Guidelines for telephone directory listings. *American Psychologist*, 1969, 24, 70-71.

11. Code of Ethics by National Association of Social Workers, Inc.

NATIONAL ASSOCIATION OF SOCIAL WORKERS, INC.
1425 H STREET, N.W., SUITE 600 ● WASHINGTON, D.C. 20005 ● PHONE
(202) 628-6800

(Adopted by the Delegate Assembly of the National Association of Social Workers, October 13, 1960, and amended April 11, 1967.)

Social work is based on humanitarian, democratic ideals. Professional social workers are dedicated to service for the welfare of mankind, to the disciplined use of a recognized body of knowledge about human beings and their interactions, and to the marshaling of community resources to promote the well-being of all without discrimination.

Social work practice is a public trust that requires of its practitioners integrity, compassion, belief in the dignity and worth of human beings, respect for individual differences, a commitment to service, and a dedication to truth. It requires mastery of a body of knowledge and skill gained through professional education and experience. It requires also recognition of the limitations of present knowledge and skill and of the services we are now equipped to give. The end sought is the performance of a service with integrity and competence.

Each member of the profession carries responsibility to maintain and improve social work service; constantly to examine, use, and increase the knowledge on which practice and social policy are based; and to develop further the philosophy and skills of the profession.

This Code of Ethics embodies certain standards of behavior for the social worker in his professional relationships with those he serves, with his colleagues, with his employing agency, with other professions, and with the community. In abiding by it, the social worker views his obligations in as wide a context as the situation requires, takes all the principles into consideration, and chooses a course of action consistent with the code's spirit and intent.

As a member of the National Association of Social Workers I commit myself to conduct my professional relationships in accord with the code and subscribe to the following statements:

■ I regard as my primary obligation the welfare of the individual or group served, which includes action for improving social conditions.

■ I will not discriminate because of race, color, religion, age, sex, or national ancestry and in my job capacity will work to prevent and eliminate such discrimination in rendering service, in work assignments, and in employment practices.

■ I give precedence to my professional responsibility over my personal interests.

■ I hold myself responsible for the quality and extent of the service I perform.

■ I respect the privacy of the people I serve.

■ I use in a responsible manner information gained in professional relationships.

■ I treat with respect the findings, views, and actions of colleagues and use appropriate channels to express judgment on these matters.

■ I practice social work within the recognized knowledge and competence of the profession.

■ I recognize my professional responsibility to add my ideas and findings to the body of social work knowledge and practice.

■ I accept responsibility to help protect the community against unethical practice by any individuals or organizations engaged in social welfare activities.

■ I stand ready to give appropriate professional service in public emergencies.

■ I distinguish clearly, in public, between my statements and actions as an individual and as a representative of an organization.

■ I support the principle that professional practice requires professional education.

■ I accept responsibility for working toward the creation and maintenance of conditions within agencies that enable social workers to conduct themselves in keeping with this code.

■ I contribute my knowledge, skills, and support to programs of human welfare.

THE PRINCIPLES OF MEDICAL ETHICS

With Annotations
Especially Applicable
to Psychiatry

1978 EDITION

Report of Chairperson, APA Ethics Committee of the approval by the APA Board of Trustees (May, 1978) of additional annotations to *The Principles of Medical Ethics with Annotations Especially Applicable to Psychiatry.*

The following has been added to annotation 10, section 9: "It is ethical to present a patient or former patient to a public gathering or to the news media only if the patient is fully informed of enduring loss of confidentiality, is competent, and consents in writing without coercion."

The following has been added to section 6: "When involved in funded research, the ethical psychiatrist will advise human subjects of the funding source, retain his or her freedom to reveal data and results, and follow all appropriate and current guidelines relative to human subject protection."

Members of the American Psychiatric Association will find additional value in the publication *Opinions and Reports of the Judicial Council,* available from the American Medical Association, 535 North Dearborn Street, Chicago, Illinois 60610; the latest revision is dated 1977.

The American Psychiatric Association
1700 18th Street N.W.
Washington, D.C. 20009
1978

The Principles of Medical Ethics
With Annotations Especially
Applicable to Psychiatry

This statement was originally approved by the Assembly and the Board of Trustees of the American Psychiatric Association at their May 5-6, 1973 meetings, upon recommendation of the Ethics Committee.[1] Additional annotations and the Procedures for Handling Complaints of Unethical Conduct were approved by the Assembly and the Board at subsequent meetings.

FOREWORD

ALL PHYSICIANS should practice in accordance with the medical code of ethics set forth in the Principles of Medical Ethics of the American Medical Association. An up-to-date expression and elaboration of these statements is found in the *Opinions and Reports of the Judicial Council* of the American Medical Association.[2] Psychiatrists are strongly advised to be familiar with these documents.[3]

However, these general guidelines have sometimes been difficult to interpret for psychiatry, so further annotations to the basic principles are offered in this document. While psychiatrists have the same goals as all physicians, there are special ethical problems in psychiatric practice that differ in coloring and degree from ethical problems in other branches of medical practice, even though the basic principles are the same. The annotations are not designed as absolutes and will be revised from time to time so as to be applicable to current practices and problems.

Following are the AMA Principles of Medical Ethics, printed in their entirety, and then each principle printed separately along with an annotation especially applicable to psychiatry.

---

[1]The committee included C.H. Hardin Branch, M.D., Chairperson, Herbert Klemmer, M.D., Robert A. Moore, M.D., Robert P. Nenno, M.D., Alex D. Pokorny, M.D., Charles D. Prudhomme, M.D., Joseph S. Skobba, M.D., and Gene Usdin, M.D. William P. Camp, M.D., and Byron A. Eliashof, M.D., were members of the subcommittee that aided in the preparation of these annotations, and William A. Bellamy, M.D., was special consultant.

[2]Judicial Council Opinions and Reports. American Medical Association. Chicago, AMA, 1977.

[3]Chapter 8, Section 1 of the By-Laws of the American Psychiatric Association states: "All members of the American Psychiatric Association shall be bound by the ethical code of the medical profession, specifically defined in the *Principles of Medical Ethics* of the American Medical Association." In interpreting the APA Constitution and By-Laws, it is the opinion of the Board of Trustees that inactive status in no way removes a physician member from responsibility to abide by the *Principles of Medical Ethics*.

PRINCIPLES OF MEDICAL ETHICS, AMERICAN MEDICAL ASSOCIATION

PREAMBLE

These principles are intended to aid physicians individually and collectively in maintaining a high level of ethical conduct. They are not laws but standards by which a physician may determine the propriety of his conduct in his relationship with patients, with colleagues, with members of allied professions, and with the public.

SECTION 1

The principal objective of the medical profession is to render service to humanity with full respect for the dignity of man. Physicians should merit the confidence of patients entrusted to their care, rendering to each a full measure of service and devotion.

SECTION 2

Physicians should strive continually to improve medical knowledge and skill, and should make available to their patients and colleagues the benefits of their professional attainments.

SECTION 3

A physician should practice a method of healing founded on a scientific basis; and he should not voluntarily associate professionally with anyone who violates this principle.

SECTION 4

The medical profession should safeguard the public and itself against physicians deficient in moral character or professional competence. Physicians should observe all laws, uphold the dignity and honor of the profession and accept its self-imposed disciplines. They should expose, without hesitation, illegal or unethical conduct of fellow members of the profession.

SECTION 5

A physician may choose whom he will serve. In an emergency, however, he should render service to the best of his ability. Having undertaken the care of a patient, he may not neglect him; and unless he has been discharged he may discontinue his services only after giving adequate notice. He should not solicit patients.

SECTION 6

A physician should not dispose of his services under terms or conditions which tend to interfere with or impair the free and complete exercise of his medical judgment and skill or tend to cause a deterioration of the quality of medical care.

SECTION 7

In the practice of medicine a physician should limit the source of his professional income to medical services actually rendered by him, or under his supervision, to his patients. His fee should be commensurate with the services rendered and the patient's ability to pay. He should neither pay nor receive a commission for referral of patients. Drugs, remedies or appliances may be dispensed or supplied by the physician provided it is in the best interest of the patient.

SECTION 8

A physician should seek consultation upon request; in doubtful or difficult cases; or whenever it appears that the quality of medical service may be enhanced thereby.

SECTION 9

A physician may not reveal the confidences entrusted to him in the course of medical attendance, or the deficiencies he may observe in the character of patients, unless he is required to do so by law or unless it becomes necessary in order to protect the welfare of the individual or of the community.

SECTION 10

The honored ideals of the medical profession imply that the responsibilities of the physician extend not only to the individual, but also to society where these responsibilities deserve his interest and participation in activities which have the purpose of improving both the health and the well-being of the individual and the community.

Principles with Annotations

Following are each of the AMA Principles of Medical Ethics printed separately along with an annotation especially applicable to psychiatry.

PREAMBLE

These principles are intended to aid physicians individually and collectively in maintaining a high level of ethical conduct. They are not laws but standards by which a physician may determine the propriety of his conduct in his relationship with patients, with colleagues, with members of allied professions, and with the public. [4]

SECTION 1

The principal objective of the medical profession is to render service to humanity with full respect for the dignity of man. Physicians should merit the confidence of patients entrusted to their care, rendering to each a full measure of service and devotion.

1. The patient may place his/her trust in his/her psychiatrist knowing that the psychiatrist's ethics and professional responsibilities preclude him/her from gratifying his/her own needs by exploiting the patient. This becomes particularly important because of the essentially private, highly personal, and sometimes intensely emotional nature of the relationship established with the psychiatrist.

2. The requirement that the physician "conduct himself with propriety in his profession and in all the actions of his life" is especially important in the case of the psychiatrist because the patient tends to model his/her behavior after that of his/her therapist by identification. Further, the necessary intensity of the therapeutic relationship may tend to activate sexual and other needs and fantasies on the part of both patient and therapist, while weakening the objectivity necessary for control. Sexual activity with a patient is unethical.

3. The psychiatrist should diligently guard against exploiting information furnished by the patient and should not use the unique position of power afforded him/her by the psychotherapeutic situation to influence the patient in any way not directly relevant to the treatment goals.

4. Physicians generally agree that the doctor-patient relationship is such a vital factor in effective treatment of the patient that preservation of optimal conditions for development of a sound working relationship between a doctor and his/her patient should take precedence over all other considerations. Professional courtesy may

---

[4]Statements in italics are taken directly from the American Medical Association's *Principles of Medical Ethics* or annotations thereto. [2]

lead to poor psychiatric care for physicians and their families because of embarrassment over the lack of a complete give-and-take contract.

SECTION 2

Physicians should strive continually to improve medical knowledge and skill, and should make available to their patients and colleagues the benefits of their professional attainments.

1. Psychiatrists are responsible for their own continuing education and should be mindful of the fact that theirs must be a lifetime of learning.

SECTION 3

A physician should practice a method of healing founded on a scientific basis and he should not voluntarily associate professionally with anyone who violates this principle.

SECTION 4

The medical profession should safeguard the public and itself against physicians deficient in moral character or professional competence. Physicians should observe all laws, uphold the dignity and honor of the profession and accept its self-imposed disciplines. They should expose, without hesitation, illegal or unethical conduct of fellow members of the profession.

1. It would seem self-evident that a psychiatrist who is a law-breaker might be ethically unsuited to practice his/her profession. When such illegal activities bear directly upon his/her practice, this would obviously be the case. However, in other instances, illegal activities such as those concerning the right to protest social injustices might not bear on either the image of the psychiatrist or the ability of the specific psychiatrist to treat his/her patient ethically and well. While no committee or board could offer prior assurance that any illegal activity would not be considered unethical, it is conceivable that an individual could violate a law without being guilty of professionally unethical behavior. Physicians lose no right of citizenship on entry into the profession of medicine.

2. A psychiatrist who regularly practices outside his/her area of professional competence should be considered unethical. Determination of professional competence should be made by peer review boards or other appropriate bodies.

3. Special consideration should be given to those psychiatrists who, because of mental illness, jeopardize the welfare of their patients and their own reputations and practices. It is ethical, even encouraged, for another psychiatrist to intercede in such situations.

4. When a member has been found to have behaved unethically by the American Psychiatric Association or one of its constituent

district branches, there should not be automatic reporting to the local authorities responsible for medical licensure, but the decision to report should be decided upon the merits of the case.[5]

5. Where not specifically prohibited by local laws governing medical practice, the practice of acupuncture by a psychiatrist is not unethical per se. The psychiatrist should have professional competence in the use of acupuncture (see Section 4, Annotation 2). Or, if he/she is supervising the use of acupuncture by non-medical individuals, he/she should provide proper medical supervision (see Section 6, Annotations 4 and 5).[6]

SECTION 5

A physician may choose whom he will serve. In an emergency, however, he should render service to the best of his ability. Having undertaken the care of a patient, he may not neglect him; and unless he has been discharged he may discontinue his services only after giving adequate notice. He should not solicit patients.

1. A psychiatrist should not be a party to any type of policy that excludes, segregates, or demeans the dignity of any patient because of ethnic origin, race, sex, creed, age, or socioeconomic status.

2. What constitutes unethical advertising, in an attempt to solicit patients, varies in different parts of the country. Local guidance should be sought from the county or state medical society. Questions that should be asked include: to whom are materials distributed, when and what is distributed, and the form in which it is distributed.[7]

SECTION 6

A physician should not dispose of his services under terms or conditions which tend to interfere with or impair the free and complete exercise of his medical judgment and skill or tend to cause a deterioration of the quality of medical care.

1. Contract practice as applied to medicine means the practice of medicine under an agreement between a physician or a group of physicians, as principals or agents, and a corporation, organization, political subdivision, or individual whereby partial or full medical services are provided for a group or class of individuals on the basis of a fee schedule, for a salary, or for a fixed rate per capita.

2. Contract practice per se is not unethical. Contract practice is unethical if it permits features or conditions that are declared unethical in these *Principles of Medical Ethics* or if the contract or any of its provisions causes deterioration of the quality of the medical services rendered.

---

[5]Approved by the Board of Trustees and the Assembly, 1975.
[6]Approved by the Board of Trustees, 1974, and the Assembly, 1975.
[7]Approved by the Board of Trustees, 1974, and the Assembly, 1975.

3. The ethical question is not the contract itself but whether or not the physician is free of unnecessary nonmedical interference. The ultimate issue is his/her freedom to offer good quality medical care.

4. In relationships between psychiatrists and practicing licensed psychologists, the physician should not delegate to the psychologist or, in fact, to any nonmedical person any matter requiring the exercise of professional medical judgment.

5. When the psychiatrist assumes a collaborative or supervisory role with another mental health worker, he/she must expend sufficient time to assure that proper care is given. It is contrary to the interests of the patient and to patient care if he/she allows himself/herself to be used as a figurehead.

6. In the practice of his/her specialty, the psychiatrist consults, associates, collaborates, or integrates his/her work with that of many professionals, including psychologists, psychometricians, social workers, alcoholism counselors, marriage counselors, public health nurses, etc. Furthermore, the nature of modern psychiatric practice extends his/her contacts to such people as teachers, juvenile and adult probation officers, attorneys, welfare workers, agency volunteers, and neighborhood aides. In referring patients for treatment, counseling, or rehabilitation to any of these practitioners, the psychiatrist should ensure that the allied professional or paraprofessional with whom he/she is dealing is a recognized member of his/her own discipline and is competent to carry out the therapeutic task required. The psychiatrist should have the same attitude toward members of the medical profession to whom he/she refers patients. Whenever he/she has reason to doubt the training, skill, or ethical qualifications of the allied professional, the psychiatrist should not refer cases to him/her.

7. Also, he/she should neither lend the endorsement of the psychiatric specialty nor refer patients to persons, groups, or treatment programs with which he/she is not familiar, especially if their work is based only on dogma and authority and not on scientific validation and replication.

8. In accord with the requirements of law and accepted medical practice, it is ethical for a physician to submit his/her work to peer review and to the ultimate authority of the medical staff executive body and the hospital administration and its governing body.

9. In case of dispute, the ethical psychiatrist has the following steps available:

a. Seek appeal from the medical staff decision to a joint conference committee, including members of the medical staff executive committee and the executive committee of the governing board. At this appeal, the ethical psychiatrist could request that outside opinions be considered.

b. Appeal to the governing body itself.

c. Appeal to state agencies regulating licensure of hospitals if, in the particular state, they concern themselves with matters of professional competency and quality of care.

d. Attempt to educate colleagues through development of research projects and data and presentations at professional meetings and in professional journals.

e. Seek redress in local courts, perhaps through an enjoining injunction against the governing body.

f. Public education as carried out by an ethical psychiatrist would not utilize appeals based solely upon emotion, but would be presented in a professional way and without any potential exploitation of patients through testimonials.[8]

SECTION 7

In the practice of medicine a physician should limit the source of his professional income to medical services actually rendered by him, or under his supervision, to his patients. His fee should be commensurate with the services rendered and the patient's ability to pay. He should neither pay nor receive a commission for referral of patients. Drugs, remedies or appliances may be dispensed or supplied by the physician provided it is in the best interests of the patient.

1. The psychiatrist may also receive income from administration, teaching, research, education, and consultation.

2. Charging for a missed appointment or for one not cancelled 24 hours in advance need not, in itself, be considered unethical if a patient is fully advised that the physician will make such a charge. The practice, however, should be resorted to infrequently and always with the utmost consideration of the patient and his circumstances.[9]

3. Psychiatric services, like all medical services, are dispensed in the context of a contractual arrangement between the patient and the treating physician. The provisions of the contractual arrangement, which are binding on the physician as well as on the patient, should be explicitly established.

4. It is ethical for the psychiatrist to make a charge for a missed appointment when this falls within the terms of the specific contractual agreement with the patient.

5. An arrangement in which a psychiatrist provides supervision or administration to other physicians or non-medical persons for a percentage of their fees or gross income is not acceptable; this would constitute fee-splitting. In a team of practitioners, or a multidisciplinary team, it is ethical for the psychiatrist to receive income for administration, research, education or consultation. This should be based upon a mutually agreed upon and set fee or salary, open to renegotiation when a change in the time demand occurs. (See also Section 6, Annotations 4, 5 and 6; and AMA Judicial Council Opinions and Reports, the section on "Public Responsibilities," VI. 6.20, 6.21, 6.22, 6.24, 6.25, 6.26, pp. 37-40).[10]

---

[8]Approved by the Board of Trustees and the Assembly, 1976.

[9]This paragraph is reprinted as an annotation to the section on "Office Practices" in AMA Judicial Council Opinions and Reports (IV.4.00, p. 15).

[10]Approved by the Board of Trustees, 1974, and the Assembly, 1975.

SECTION 8

A physician should seek consultation upon request; in doubtful or difficult cases; or whenever it appears that the quality of the medical service may be enhanced thereby.

1. The psychiatrist should agree to the request of a patient for consultation or to such a request from the family of an incompetent or minor patient. The psychiatrist may suggest possible consultants, but the patient or family should be given free choice of the consultant. If the psychiatrist disapproves of the professional qualifications of the consultant or if there is a difference of opinion that the primary therapist cannot resolve he/she may, after suitable notice, withdraw from the case. If this disagreement occurs within an institution or agency framework, the differences should be resolved by the mediation or arbitration of higher professional authority within the institution or agency.

SECTION 9

A physician may not reveal the confidences entrusted to him in the course of medical attendance, or the deficiencies he may observe in the character of patients, unless he is required to do so by law or unless it becomes necessary in order to protect the welfare of the individual or of the community.

1. Psychiatric records, including even the identification of a person as a patient, must be protected with extreme care. Confidentiality is essential to psychiatric treatment. This is based in part on the special nature of psychiatric therapy as well as on the traditional ethical relationship between physician and patient. Growing concern regarding the civil rights of patients and the possible adverse effects of computerization, duplication equipment, and data banks makes the dissemination of confidential information an increasing hazard. Because of the sensitive and private nature of the information with which the psychiatrist deals, he/she must be circumspect in the information that he/she chooses to disclose to others about a patient. The welfare of the patient must be a continuing consideration.

2. A psychiatrist may release confidential information only with the authorization of the patient or under proper legal compulsion. The continuing duty of the psychiatrist to protect the patient includes fully apprising him/her of the connotations of waiving the privilege of privacy. This may become an issue when the patient is being investigated by a government agency, is applying for a position, or is involved in legal action. The same principles apply to the release of information concerning treatment to medical departments of government agencies, business organizations, labor unions, and insurance companies. Information gained in confidence about patients seen in student health services should not be released without the student's explicit permission.

3. Clinical and other materials used in teaching and writing must be adequately disguised in order to preserve the anonymity of the individuals involved.

4. The ethical responsibility of maintaining confidentiality holds equally for the consultations in which the patient may not have been present and in which the consultee was not a physician. In such instances, the physician consultant should alert the consultee to his/her duty of confidentiality.

5. Ethically the psychiatrist may disclose only that information which is immediately relevant to a given situation. He/she should avoid offering speculation as fact. Sensitive information such as an individual's sexual orientation or fantasy material is usually unnecessary.

6. Psychiatrists are often asked to examine individuals for security purposes, to determine suitability for various jobs, and to determine legal competence. The psychiatrist must fully describe the nature and purpose and lack of confidentiality of the examination to the examinee at the beginning of the examination.

7. Psychiatrists at times may find it necessary, in order to protect the patient or the community from imminent danger, to reveal confidential information disclosed by the patient.

8. Careful judgment must be exercised by the psychiatrist in order to include, when appropriate, the parents or guardian in the treatment of a minor. At the same time the psychiatrist must assure the minor proper confidentiality.

9. When the psychiatrist is ordered by the court to reveal the confidences entrusted to him/her by patients he/she may comply or he/she may ethically hold the right to dissent within the framework of the law. When the psychiatrist is in doubt, the right of the patient to confidentiality and, by extension, to unimpaired treatment, should be given priority. The psychiatrist should reserve the right to raise the question of adequate need for disclosure. In the event that the necessity for legal disclosure is demonstrated by the court, the psychiatrist may request the right to disclosure of only that information which is relevant to the legal question at hand.

10. With regard for the person's dignity and privacy and with truly informed consent, it is ethical to present a patient to a scientific gathering, if the confidentiality of the presentation is understood and accepted by the audience.[11]

SECTION 10

The honored ideals of the medical profession imply that the responsibilities of the physician extend not only to the individual, but also to society where these responsibilities deserve his interest and participation in activities which have the purpose of improving both the health and the well-being of the individual and the community.

---

[11]Approved by the Board of Trustees and the Assembly, 1975.

1. Psychiatrists should foster the cooperation of those legitimately concerned with the medical, psychological, social, and legal aspects of mental health and illness. Psychiatrists are encouraged to serve society by advising and consulting with the executive, legislative, and judiciary branches of the government. A psychiatrist should clarify whether he/she speaks as an individual or as a representative of an organization. Furthermore, psychiatrists should avoid cloaking their public statements with the authority of the profession (e.g., "Psychiatrists know that. . .").

2. Psychiatrists may interpret and share with the public their expertise in the various psychosocial issues that may affect mental health and illness. Psychiatrists should always be mindful of their separate roles as dedicated citizens and as experts in psychological medicine.

3. On occasion psychiatrists are asked for an opinion about an individual who is in the light of public attention, or who has disclosed information about himself through public media. It is unethical for a psychiatrist to offer a professional opinion unless he/she has conducted an examination and has been granted proper authorization for such a statement.

4. The psychiatrist may only permit his/her certification to be used for the involuntary treatment of any person following his/her personal examination of that person. To do so, he/she must find that the person, because of mental illness, cannot form a judgment as to what is in his/her own best interests and without which treatment substantial impairment is likely to occur to the person or others.[12]

---

[12]Approved by the Executive Committee and the Assembly, 1977.

Procedures for Handling Complaints of Unethical Conduct[13]

A complaint concerning the behavior of a member of this Association shall be in writing, signed by the complainant, and filed with the Secretary. The Secretary shall refer it to the appropriate District Branch for investigation and action. The Secretary shall notify the accused member of the receipt of such a complaint and that it has been forwarded to the member's local District Branch and shall inform the accused member of his or her right to appeal any forthcoming action to the Board. The District Branch may appeal to the Board for relief from responsibility for considering any complaint. The member against whom the complaint was brought shall have the right of appeal to the Board for reconsideration of the decision of the District Branch.[14]

As noted above, a complaint must be written, must be signed by the complainant, and must be filed with the Secretary of the Association.

Procedure A. Allegation Received by District Branch

I.   District Branch:

    A. Receives signed communication alleging or inferring unethical conduct.

    B. Determines the membership status of the potential defendant.

    C. Determines if allegation or inference constitutes a complaint of unethical conduct as defined in the PRINCIPLES OF MEDICAL ETHICS WITH ANNOTATIONS ESPECIALLY APPLICABLE TO PSYCHIATRY — that is, does the allegation or inference merit an investigation, and, if so, files a copy of the complaint with the Secretary of the American Psychiatric Association.

II. Secretary of the American Psychiatric Association:

    A. Receives written and signed copy of the complaint from the District Branch and refers complaint back to the Branch for investigation.

    B. Notifies the accused member that a copy of a complaint has been received and filed, that the investigation will be conducted by the District Branch and of the member's right to appeal a negative decision to the Board of Trustees of the American Psychiatric Association.

---

[13]Approved by the Executive Committee and the Assembly, 1975; revision approved by the Board of Trustees and the Assembly, 1977.
[14]Chapter 10, Section 1, By-Laws, American Psychiatric Association, 1977 revision.

III. District Branch:

A. Upon receiving complaint from the Secretary of the American Psychiatric Association, notifies the accused member of the complaint, who made the complaint, relates the complaint to the appropriate Section(s) of the PRINCIPLES OF MEDICAL ETHICS WITH ANNOTATIONS ESPECIALLY APPLICABLE TO PSYCHIATRY, informs the accused member of his/her right to be advised and represented by legal counsel, and forward to him/her a copy of the complaint, these PROCEDURES, the PRINCIPLES OF MEDICAL ETHICS WITH ANNOTATIONS ESPECIALLY APPLICABLE TO PSYCHIATRY, all addenda to the PROCEDURES and PRINCIPLES, and a copy of the Constitution and By-Laws of the American Psychiatric Association.

B. Notifies complainant that the complaint has been received, will be investigated, of his/her right to legal counsel during the investigation, and that he/she will be informed of the decision of the District Branch.

C. Refers the complaint to the District Branch Ethics Committee or whatever body serves that function for investigation and recommendations for action to the Council of the District Branch.

D. Ethics Committee or whatever body serves that function investigates the complaint, permitting both the defendant and complainant to be heard. If the complainant is expected to produce evidence, he/she should be so advised in writing.

E. May refer the complaint to the American Psychiatric Association for investigation under unusual circumstances and then PROCEDURE B would be followed, with the APA Ethics Committee conducting the investigation. Unusual circumstances would include, but not be limited to, conflicts of interest, interested parties from different parts of the country, or a complaint of significant national importance.

F. The Council of the District Branch, upon receiving the recommendation for action, determines:

1. Either that the complaint is without merit and dismisses it;

2. Or, that the complaint has been sustained and the defendant shall be subject to one of the following penalties:

   a. admonishment
   b. reprimand

        c. suspension from membership for a specific period of time

        d. expulsion from the District Branch.

    G. Notifies the Secretary of the American Psychiatric Association of the procedures followed, the Section under which the complaint was filed, and the action taken.

IV.   Secretary of the American Psychiatric Association:

    A. Receives the report of the District Branch.

    B. Sends the report to the Ethics Committee of the American Psychiatric Association.

V.   Ethics Committee of the American Psychiatric Association:

    A. Reviews the procedures followed by the District Branch.

    B. Obtains additional information from the District Branch about procedures if necessary.

    C. Reports to the Board of Trustees on the procedures followed and the action taken.

VI.   Board of Trustees of the American Psychiatric Association:

    A. On recommendation of the Ethics Committee of the American Psychiatric Association:

        1. Approves that proper procedures have been followed. If not approved, the District Branch is directed to complete this investigation properly following the procedures.

        2. Receives the report of action taken.

        3. Orders the action taken be kept in a confidential file, listed by initial of the defendant only.

        4. When expulsion from the District Branch is the action, notifies the defendant of his expulsion from the American Psychiatric Association and his right of appeal.

    B. Instructs the Secretary of the American Psychiatric Association to notify the District Branch whether or not proper procedures have been followed.

VII. District Branch:

    A. Notifies the accused member of action taken and his/her rights of appeal.

    B. Notifies complainant of action taken after avenues of appeal to the American Psychiatric Association have been exhausted or waived.

VIII. Appeal Procedure:

    A. Within 30 days of receipt of notice of action by the District Branch (and the Board of Trustees in case of expulsion), the defendant files written notice of his/her appeal with the Secretary of the American Psychiatric Association.

    B. The Secretary of the American Psychiatric Association notifies the District Branch of the appeal and asks them to submit all information in their possession. The defendant is asked to submit the justification for his/her appeal and any information which he/she has which would support his/her appeal.

    C. This information is submitted to the APA Ethics Committee. The defendant, with thirty (30) days' written notice, has the right to personal appearance, accompanied by legal counsel if he/she wishes, before the APA Ethics Committee. The APA Ethics Committee has the right to request the defendant and/or complainant to appear, with legal counsel if desired by either. (See Procedure B.IV.D.).

Procedure B. Allegations Received by The American Psychiatric Asscociation

I.   Secretary of the American Psychiatric Association:

    A. Receives signed communication alleging or inferring unethical conduct.

    B. Determines the membership status of the potential defendant.

    C. Determines if allegation or inference constitutes a complaint of unethical conduct as defined in the PRINCIPLES OF MEDICAL ETHICS WITH ANNOTATIONS ESPECIALLY APPLICABLE TO PSYCHIATRY — that is, does the allegation or inference merit an investigation.

    D. Notifies the accused member of the complaint, who made the complaint, relates the complaint to the appropriate Section(s) of the PRINCIPLES OF MEDICAL ETHICS WITH ANNOTATIONS ESPECIALLY APPLICABLE TO PSYCHIATRY, informs the accused member of his/her right to be advised and represented by legal counsel, and forwards to him/her a copy of the complaint, these PROCEDURES, the PRINCIPLES OF MEDICAL ETHICS WITH ANNOTATIONS ESPECIALLY APPLICABLE TO PSYCHIATRY, all addenda to the PROCEDURES AND PRINCIPLES, and a copy of the Constitution and By-Laws of the American Psychiatric Association.

    E. Notifies complainant that complaint has been received, that an investigation will be conducted by the District

Branch (or APA Ethics Committee), advises him/her of his/her right to legal counsel during the investigation, and that he/she will be informed of the decision.

F. Sends complaint to the District Branch for investigation with information to the APA Ethics Committee.

II. District Branch:

A. Accepts the responsibility and assigns investigation to its Ethics Committee or whatever body acts in that capacity (and the Committee follows Procedures A.I.); recommendations from that body are made to the Council of the District Branch.

B. The Council of the District Branch determines:

1. Either that the complaint is without merit and dismisses it;

2. Or, that the complaint has been sustained and the defendant shall be subject to one of the following penalties:

a. admonishment
b. reprimand
c. suspension from membership for a specific period of time
d. expulsion from the District Branch.

C. The Council of the District Branch notifies the Secretary of the American Psychiatric Association of the procedures followed and the action recommended.

III. Secretary of the American Psychiatric Association:

A. Reviews the procedures and recommendations of the District Branch.

B. Sends the report to the APA Ethics Committee.

IV. Ethics Committee of the American Psychiatric Association:

A. Reviews the procedures and recommendations of the District Branch.

B. Obtains additional information from the District Branch about procedures and recommendations if necessary.

C. Reports to the APA Board of Trustees on the procedures followed and actions recommended.

D. When the APA Ethics Committee is the original investigating body:

1. The Ethics Committee may request two Fellows of the American Psychiatric Association residing in the same area as the complainant and defendant to serve as in-

vestigators. These investigators may interview the parties and gather other pertinent information which they will submit to the Ethics Committee. If the complainant is expected to produce evidence, he/she should be so advised in writing.

2. Because of possible distances involved, the defendant and complainant shall be given thirty (30) days' notice in writing of the time and place of the meeting of the Ethics Committee.

3. The defendant and complainant shall have the right to appear and to legal counsel.

4. The Ethics Committee makes its recommendation to the Board of Trustees.

V. Board of Trustees of the American Psychiatric Association:

A. On recommendation of the APA Ethics Committee:

1. Approves that proper procedures have been followed. If not approved, the District Branch (or the Ethics Committee if the investigating body) is directed to complete their investigation properly following the procedures.

2. Approves, disapproves, or modifies the action recommended by the District Branch (or the Ethics Committee if the investigating body). In case of expulsion, a two-thirds (2/3) vote of the Board of Trustees is required.

3. Notifies the complainant after avenues of appeal have been exhausted or waived, and the defendant and the District Branch of the action taken. The defendant is again advised of his/her right to appeal and to be represented by legal counsel.

4. Orders the action taken be kept in a confidential file, listed by initial of the defendant only.

5. In the case of expulsion, the member is also expelled from the District Branch.

VI. Appeal Procedure:

A. Within thirty (30) days of receipt of action by the APA Board of Trustees, the defendant files written notice with the Secretary of the American Psychiatric Association of his/her appeal.

B. Expelled members shall be denied all membership privileges pending the appeal.

C. All other penalties shall be suspended pending the appeal.

D. The appeal shall be heard at the next Annual Meeting of the American Psychiatric Association at a session attended only by voting members and the necessary secretarial staff and legal counsel as selected by the President.

E. The defendant shall have the right to be heard, present his/her evidence, and be represented by legal counsel.

F. Presentation of evidence and arguments for the American Psychiatric Association shall be made by the President or a member of his choice.

G. A two-thirds (2/3) vote of those present by secret written ballot shall be required to reverse the action of the Board of Trustees, leading to a modified action or dismissal of the charges.

OUTLINE REPORT
RESULTS OF ETHICS COMPLAINT INVESTIGATION

District Branch: _____

Initials of Complainant & Defendant: _____

Complaint:

   Section: _____

   Brief Description: _____

_____

_____

_____

_____

_____

Initiated at:

   District Branch (Procedure A): _____

   APA (Procedure B): _____

Preliminary review shows complaint to be without sufficient merit
for further investigation: _____

Complainant advised and action taken:

   Right to be heard: _____

   Right to counsel: _____

Defendant advised and action taken: _____

   Right to be heard: _____

   Right of confrontation of complainant: _____

     (At the discretion of the district branch)

   Right to counsel: _____

   Right of appeal: _____

Findings and brief justification: _____

_____

_____

_____

_____

_____

_____

Recommended Action: _____

   Admonishment: _____

   Reprimand: _____

   Suspension: _____

   Expulsion: _____

     Other actions modifying above: _____

       Signed _____ Date _____

       Address _____

       Office _____

INDEX

Index

Index

Index